Ninja Foodi 2-Basket Air Fryer Cookbook for Beginners 2024

Super Easy, Delicious Air Fryer Recipes to Enjoy Frying Without Getting Fat and Healthier Eating Habits, Include Dehydrate, Roast and More

Sheila R. Donato

Copyright © 2024 by Sheila R. Donato

All rights reserved.

Welcome to Sheila R. Donato's Ninja Foodi 2-Basket Air Fryer Cookbook for Beginners 2024. We're thrilled to have you embark on this culinary journey with us. Before you dive into these delectable recipes, please take a moment to review our copyright statement and disclaimer, which outline the terms and conditions of using this recipe book.

This recipe book and its contents are protected by copyright law. We've poured our heart and soul into crafting these recipes and the accompanying content. We kindly request that you respect our efforts by not reproducing, storing, or distributing any part of this book in any form without our prior written consent.

By using this recipe book, you agree to abide by the terms outlined in this copyright statement and disclaimer.

While we encourage you to share your culinary experiences with friends and family, we ask that you do so within the boundaries of personal, non-commercial use. Brief quotations for critical reviews and similar non-commercial purposes are permitted, but please ensure that our work is acknowledged.

CONTENTS

INTRODUCTION 7
    What is a Dual Zone Air Fryer? 8
    Ingredient Cooking Chart 9
    How To Air Fry: Air Fryer Tips For Beginners 9
    How to Clean an Air Fryer? 10

Breakfast Recipes 11

Honey Banana Oatmeal 11	Sweet Potato Sausage Hash 17
Healthy Oatmeal Muffins 11	Egg With Baby Spinach 17
Yellow Potatoes With Eggs 11	Morning Egg Rolls 17
Cornbread 11	Sausage & Butternut Squash 18
Quiche Breakfast Peppers 12	Cheesy Baked Eggs 18
Lemon-cream Cheese Danishes Cherry Danishes 12	Hash Browns 18
Sweet Potato Hash 13	Bagels 19
Sausage Hash And Baked Eggs 13	Egg And Avocado In The Ninja Foodi 19
Banana Muffins 13	Banana And Raisins Muffins 19
Breakfast Stuffed Peppers 14	Breakfast Sausage Omelet 20
Sweet Potatoes Hash 14	Sausage Breakfast Casserole 20
Blueberry Coffee Cake And Maple Sausage Patties 14	Crispy Hash Browns 20
Breakfast Frittata 15	Turkey Ham Muffins 20
Air Fried Sausage 15	Brussels Sprouts Potato Hash 21
Perfect Cinnamon Toast 15	Glazed Apple Fritters Glazed Peach Fritters 21
Pepper Egg Cups 15	Vanilla Strawberry Doughnuts 22
Buttermilk Biscuits With Roasted Stone Fruit Compote 16	Cinnamon Apple French Toast 22
Egg White Muffins 16	Breakfast Bacon 22

Snacks And Appetizers Recipes 23

Peppered Asparagus 23	Blueberries Muffins 27
Cauliflower Gnocchi 23	Zucchini Chips 28
Bacon Wrapped Tater Tots 23	Tofu Veggie Meatballs 28
Fried Halloumi Cheese 23	Stuffed Bell Peppers 28
Spicy Chicken Tenders 24	Fried Ravioli 28
Chicken Crescent Wraps 24	Tater Tots 29
Fried Pickles 24	Mac And Cheese Balls 29
Cheddar Quiche 24	Crispy Plantain Chips 29
Crab Cakes 25	Fried Cheese 30
Beef Jerky Pineapple Jerky 25	Potato Chips 30
Strawberries And Walnuts Muffins 25	"fried" Ravioli With Zesty Marinara 30
Parmesan French Fries 26	Mozzarella Balls 31
Onion Rings 26	Chili-lime Crispy Chickpeas Pizza-seasoned Crispy Chickpeas 31
Healthy Spinach Balls 26	Tasty Sweet Potato Wedges 31
Miso-glazed Shishito Peppers Charred Lemon Shishito Peppers 27	Kale Potato Nuggets 32
Sweet Bites 27	Crab Rangoon Dip With Crispy Wonton Strips 32

Cinnamon Sugar Chickpeas 32
Dried Apple Chips Dried Banana Chips 33
Parmesan Crush Chicken 33
Roasted Tomato Bruschetta With Toasty Garlic Bread .. 33

Fish And Seafood Recipes 34

Breaded Scallops 34
Seafood Shrimp Omelet 34
Crispy Catfish 35
Codfish With Herb Vinaigrette 35
Bang Bang Shrimp With Roasted Bok Choy 35
Fried Tilapia 36
Spicy Salmon Fillets 36
Salmon Patties 36
Foil Packet Salmon 37
Lemon Pepper Fish Fillets 37
Buttered Mahi-mahi 37
Crusted Shrimp 37
Fish And Chips 38
Cajun Scallops 38
Bacon-wrapped Shrimp 38
Salmon Nuggets 39
Tilapia With Mojo And Crispy Plantains 39
Lemon Pepper Salmon With Asparagus 40
Shrimp With Lemon And Pepper 40
Flavorful Salmon With Green Beans 40
Scallops With Greens 40
Herb Tuna Patties 41
Honey Teriyaki Tilapia 41
Bang Bang Shrimp 41
Garlic Butter Salmon 42
Salmon With Coconut 42
Frozen Breaded Fish Fillet 42
Stuffed Mushrooms With Crab 42
Smoked Salmon 43
Herb Lemon Mussels 43
Shrimp Po'boys With Sweet Potato Fries 43
Crusted Cod 44
Beer Battered Fish Fillet 44
Furikake Salmon 45
Fish Tacos 45
Chili Lime Tilapia 45

Vegetables And Sides Recipes 46

Air-fried Tofu Cutlets With Cacio E Pepe Brussels
Sprouts 46
Broccoli, Squash, & Pepper 46
Jerk Tofu With Roasted Cabbage 46
Green Beans With Baked Potatoes 47
Rosemary Asparagus & Potatoes 47
Stuffed Sweet Potatoes 47
Air Fried Okra 48
Healthy Air Fried Veggies 48
Spanakopita Rolls With Mediterranean Vegetable Salad 48
Lime Glazed Tofu 49
Quinoa Patties 49
Veggie Burgers With "fried" Onion Rings 50
Acorn Squash Slices 51
Sweet Potatoes & Brussels Sprouts 51
Mixed Air Fry Veggies 51
Bacon Wrapped Corn Cob 51
Zucchini Cakes 52
Green Tomato Stacks 52
Fried Artichoke Hearts 52
Air-fried Radishes 53
Curly Fries 53
Bacon Potato Patties 53
Garlic-rosemary Brussels Sprouts 54
Hasselback Potatoes 54
Buffalo Seitan With Crispy Zucchini Noodles 54
Fried Avocado Tacos 55
Fried Patty Pan Squash 55
Delicious Potatoes & Carrots 55
Garlic Potato Wedges In Air Fryer 56
Fried Asparagus 56
Garlic-herb Fried Squash 56
Bbq Corn 57
Fried Olives 57
Mushroom Roll-ups 57
Kale And Spinach Chips 57
Potatoes & Beans 58

Beef, Pork, And Lamb Recipes 58

- Mustard Rubbed Lamb Chops 58
- Lamb Chops With Dijon Garlic 59
- Gochujang Brisket 59
- Beef And Bean Taquitos With Mexican Rice 59
- Easy Breaded Pork Chops 60
- Steak In Air Fry 60
- Garlic Butter Steaks 60
- Air Fryer Meatloaves 61
- Meatloaf 61
- Turkey And Beef Meatballs 61
- Pork With Green Beans And Potatoes 62
- Meatballs 62
- Bell Peppers With Sausages 62
- Italian-style Meatballs With Garlicky Roasted Broccoli 63
- Bacon Wrapped Pork Tenderloin 63
- Balsamic Steak Tips With Roasted Asparagus And Mushroom Medley 63
- Beef Cheeseburgers 64
- Tender Pork Chops 64
- Pork Chops With Brussels Sprouts 64
- Cinnamon-apple Pork Chops 65
- Lamb Shank With Mushroom Sauce 65
- Juicy Pork Chops 65
- Chinese Bbq Pork 66
- Pork Chops With Apples 66
- Garlic-rosemary Pork Loin With Scalloped Potatoes And Cauliflower 66
- Korean Bbq Beef 67
- Tasty Pork Skewers 67
- Glazed Steak Recipe 68
- Pork Chops And Potatoes 68
- Beef Ribs I 68
- Paprika Pork Chops 68
- Sausage Meatballs 69
- Breaded Pork Chops 69
- Roast Beef 69
- Chipotle Beef 70
- Steak Bites With Cowboy Butter 70

Poultry Recipes 71

- Buttermilk Fried Chicken 71
- Ranch Turkey Tenders With Roasted Vegetable Salad .. 71
- Spicy Chicken Sandwiches With "fried" Pickles 72
- Chicken Parmesan With Roasted Lemon-parmesan Broccoli 72
- Balsamic Duck Breast 73
- Wings With Corn On The Cob 73
- Spicy Chicken Wings 73
- Spice-rubbed Chicken Pieces 74
- Glazed Thighs With French Fries 74
- Sweet-and-sour Chicken With Pineapple Cauliflower Rice 74
- Asian Chicken 75
- Sweet And Spicy Carrots With Chicken Thighs .. 75
- Marinated Chicken Legs 75
- Thai Curry Chicken Kabobs 76
- Bang-bang Chicken 76
- Almond Chicken 76
- Cheddar-stuffed Chicken 76
- Goat Cheese–stuffed Chicken Breast With Broiled Zucchini And Cherry Tomatoes 77
- Air-fried Turkey Breast With Roasted Green Bean Casserole 77
- Chicken Drumettes 78
- Chicken Ranch Wraps 78
- Easy Chicken Thighs 78
- Greek Chicken Meatballs 79
- Coconut Chicken Tenders With Broiled Utica Greens ... 79
- Roasted Garlic Chicken Pizza With Cauliflower "wings" 80
- Cajun Chicken With Vegetables 80
- "fried" Chicken With Warm Baked Potato Salad 80
- Cornish Hen With Asparagus 81
- Chicken Kebabs 81
- Chicken Vegetable Skewers 82
- Chicken And Broccoli 82
- Chicken & Broccoli 82
- Chicken And Potatoes 83
- Crispy Sesame Chicken 83
- Lemon Chicken Thighs 83
- Chicken Breast Strips 84

Desserts Recipes 85

Fried Dough With Roasted Strawberries 85	Apple Crisp 91
Baked Apples 85	Dehydrated Peaches 92
Banana Spring Rolls With Hot Fudge Dip 85	Pumpkin Muffins With Cinnamon 92
Monkey Bread 86	Cinnamon Bread Twists 92
Fudge Brownies 86	Chocó Lava Cake 92
Chocolate Chip Cake 87	Moist Chocolate Espresso Muffins 93
Chocolate Cookies 87	Walnut Baklava Bites Pistachio Baklava Bites 93
Mini Strawberry And Cream Pies 87	Grilled Peaches 93
Bread Pudding 87	Apple Crumble Peach Crumble 94
Pumpkin Hand Pies Blueberry Hand Pies 88	Churros 94
Zesty Cranberry Scones 88	Apple Hand Pies 94
Delicious Apple Fritters 89	Air Fryer Sweet Twists 95
Air Fried Bananas 89	Dessert Empanadas 95
Strawberry Shortcake 89	Lava Cake 96
"air-fried" Oreos Apple Fries 89	Apple Nutmeg Flautas 96
Pumpkin Muffins 90	Jelly Donuts 96
Mocha Pudding Cake Vanilla Pudding Cake 90	Cinnamon Sugar Dessert Fries 97
Healthy Semolina Pudding 91	S'mores Dip With Cinnamon-sugar Tortillas 97

APPENDIX A: Measurement 98

APPENDIX B: Recipes Index 100

INTRODUCTION

In the bustling world of modern cooking, where convenience and versatility are cherished as highly as flavor and nutrition, one kitchen appliance has made a significant impact: the Ninja Foodi 2-Basket Air Fryer. For those who relish the joy of creating delectable meals without the hassle of multiple cooking gadgets and extensive cleanup, the Ninja Foodi 2-Basket Air Fryer stands as an indispensable culinary companion. It's a game-changer, a kitchen revolution, and the key to unlocking a world of limitless culinary possibilities, all in one compact and efficient device.

As you hold this cookbook in your hands, you're about to embark on an exciting journey of culinary exploration, guided by the expertise of a passionate and experienced chef, Sheila R. Donato. Sheila has spent years crafting and perfecting recipes that not only harness the remarkable capabilities of the Ninja Foodi 2-Basket Air Fryer but also satisfy the cravings and desires of food enthusiasts from all walks of life. Her journey began with a love for cooking, a curiosity for innovation, and a keen sense of how to make every meal a memorable experience.

In the "Ninja Foodi 2-Basket Air Fryer Cookbook," Sheila shares her culinary wisdom, creativity, and a treasure trove of recipes that showcase the incredible potential of this remarkable kitchen appliance. Whether you are a seasoned home chef or someone taking their first steps into the world of cooking, Sheila's cookbook provides a roadmap to transforming ordinary ingredients into extraordinary dishes, effortlessly and with minimal fuss.

Moreover, this cookbook goes beyond just recipes. Sheila shares valuable tips, techniques, and insights into making the most of your Ninja Foodi 2-Basket Air Fryer, so you can confidently create culinary masterpieces that will impress both family and friends. From selecting the right cooking temperatures and times to maximizing the potential of dual-zone cooking, you'll find comprehensive guidance that will transform you into a culinary maestro in your own kitchen.

What is a Dual Zone Air Fryer?

Before we get started, there's a good chance you already have an air fryer, which is why you're here, but just in case, let's take a look at what this amazing kitchen gadget actually does!

An air fryer is an easy and healthy way to cook food instead of frying or sautéing it.

It cooks food by circulating hot air around the food without using any oil!

Air fryers are great for making snacks, side dishes, entrees, desserts ...... and desserts! It's an easy way to reduce fat intake without sacrificing flavor or texture.

Air fryers also cook food quickly, making them perfect for busy families who don't want to spend a long time preparing and cooking every day.

Another benefit is that air fryers don't take up much space, which is helpful if you have limited bench space or cupboard storage!

And the best feature of a dual zone air fryer is that it allows you to cook two dishes at the same time, a huge time saver!

Ingredient Cooking Chart

Ingredient	Temperature (°F or °C)	Time (minutes)	Notes/Instructions
Chicken Wings	360°F (182°C)	20-25	Preheat the air fryer. Flip halfway for even cooking.
French Fries	380°F (193°C)	15-20	Shake the basket halfway through for crispiness.
Salmon Fillet	380°F (193°C)	10-12	Brush with olive oil, season, and preheat the air fryer.
Vegetable Fritters	350°F (177°C)	12-15	Use a light coating of oil for a crispy texture.
Mozzarella Sticks	380°F (193°C)	6-8	Freeze for 1 hour before air frying for best results.
Pork Chops	360°F (182°C)	12-15	Season and preheat the air fryer for even cooking.
Shrimp	400°F (204°C)	5-7	Lightly coat with oil and season before cooking.

How To Air Fry: Air Fryer Tips For Beginners

Air fryers are so easy to use. Just make sure you follow the instructions to get started. Here are a few of our best tips for getting started, so you can uplevel your air frying game:

- Easy Air Fryer Recipes for Beginners & Tips To Get Started

- Do not overcrowd your air fryer basket. This may mean cooking your food in batches, however, this is better than having your food unevenly cooked.

- Flip foods halfway through the cooking time so that they cook evenly just as you would if you were grilling or frying.

- Air fryers cook food more quickly than an oven or stovetop, so keep a regular eye on the time and temperature to prevent overcooking your food.

- While preheating isn't necessary when air frying food, it can help cook food more evenly. If your air fryer does not have a pre-heat option, just run it for 2-3 minutes at the temperature you plan to cook with before starting.

- If you're cooking meat, be mindful of the doneness so that it doesn't overcook or undercook!

How to Clean an Air Fryer?

Cleaning an air fryer is essential to maintain its performance, prevent odors, and ensure the longevity of the appliance.

Materials Needed:

Dishwashing liquid or mild detergent

Warm water

Non-abrasive sponge or cloth

Soft brush or toothbrush

Soft, dry cloth or paper towels

Cleaning the Air Fryer Basket and Pan:

Cool Down the Air Fryer: Ensure that the air fryer has cooled down completely before attempting to clean it. This prevents the risk of burns.

Remove the Basket and Pan: Carefully pull out the air fryer basket and pan from the appliance. Empty any food residue or crumbs into the trash.

Soak in Warm, Soapy Water: Fill a sink or basin with warm water and add a few drops of dishwashing liquid or mild detergent. Submerge the basket and pan in the soapy water and let them soak for 10-15 minutes.

Clean with a Soft Sponge: Gently scrub the basket and pan with a non-abrasive sponge or cloth to remove any remaining food particles or grease. Be cautious not to scratch the non-stick coating.

Rinse and Dry: Rinse the basket and pan thoroughly with clean water to remove any soap residue. Use a soft, dry cloth or paper towels to wipe them dry.

Additional Tips:

1. Avoid using abrasive scouring pads, steel wool, or harsh chemicals, as they can damage the non-stick coating and exterior finish.

2. Regular cleaning after each use is recommended to prevent the buildup of stubborn residues.

3. If there are persistent, burnt-on stains or residue, you can make a paste using baking soda and water. Apply the paste to the affected areas, let it sit for a few minutes, and then gently scrub with a soft sponge before rinsing and drying.

4. Some air fryer components, such as the basket and pan, may be dishwasher safe. Check the manufacturer's instructions to confirm if these parts are dishwasher-friendly.

Breakfast Recipes

Honey Banana Oatmeal

Servings: 4
Cooking Time: 8 Minutes
Ingredients:
- 2 eggs
- 2 tbsp honey
- 1 tsp vanilla
- 45g quick oats
- 73ml milk
- 30g Greek yoghurt
- 219g banana, mashed

Directions:
1. In a bowl, mix eggs, milk, yoghurt, honey, vanilla, oats, and mashed banana until well combined.
2. Pour batter into the four greased ramekins.
3. Insert a crisper plate in the Ninja Foodi air fryer baskets.
4. Place ramekins in both baskets.
5. Select zone 1 then select "air fry" mode and set the temperature to 390 degrees F for 8 minutes. Press "match" to match zone 2 settings to zone 1. Press "start/stop" to begin.

Nutrition Info:
- (Per serving) Calories 228 | Fat 4.6g |Sodium 42mg | Carbs 40.4g | Fiber 4.2g | Sugar 16.1g | Protein 7.7g

Healthy Oatmeal Muffins

Servings: 6
Cooking Time: 17 Minutes
Ingredients:
- 1 egg
- ¼ tsp ground ginger
- 1 tsp ground cinnamon
- ½ tsp baking soda
- ½ tsp baking powder
- 55g brown sugar
- ½ tsp vanilla
- 2 tbsp butter, melted
- 125g applesauce
- 61ml milk
- 68gm whole wheat flour
- 100gm quick oats
- Pinch of salt

Directions:
1. In a mixing bowl, mix together all dry the ingredients.
2. In a separate bowl, add the remaining ingredients and mix well.
3. Add the dry ingredients mixture into the wet mixture and mix until well combined.
4. Pour the batter into the silicone muffin moulds.
5. Insert a crisper plate in the Ninja Foodi air fryer baskets.
6. Place muffin moulds in both baskets.
7. Select zone 1 then select "bake" mode and set the temperature to 390 degrees F for 17 minutes. Press "start/stop" to begin.

Nutrition Info:
- (Per serving) Calories 173 | Fat 5.8g |Sodium 177mg | Carbs 26.6g | Fiber 2.1g | Sugar 8.7g | Protein 4.2g

Yellow Potatoes With Eggs

Servings:2
Cooking Time:35
Ingredients:
- 1 pound of Dutch yellow potatoes, quartered
- 1 red bell pepper, chopped
- Salt and black pepper, to taste
- 1 green bell pepper, chopped
- 2 teaspoons of olive oil
- 2 teaspoons of garlic powder
- 1 teaspoon of onion powder
- 1 egg
- ¼ teaspoon of butter

Directions:
1. Toss together diced potatoes, green pepper, red pepper, salt, black pepper, and olive oil along with garlic powder and onion powder.
2. Put in the zone 1 basket of the air fryer.
3. Take ramekin and grease it with oil spray.
4. Whisk egg in a bowl and add salt and pepper along with ½ teaspoon of butter.
5. Pour egg into a ramekin and place it in a zone 2 basket.
6. Now start cooking and set a timer for zone 1 basket to 30-35 minutes at 400 degrees at AIR FRY mode.
7. Now for zone 2, set it on AIR FRY mode at 350 degrees F for 8-10 minutes.
8. Press the Smart finish button and press start, it will finish both at the same time.
9. Once done, serve and enjoy.

Nutrition Info:
- (Per serving) Calories252 | Fat7.5g | Sodium 37mg | Carbs 40g | Fiber3.9g | Sugar 7g | Protein 6.7g

Cornbread

Servings: 6
Cooking Time: 15 Minutes
Ingredients:
- 1 cup cornmeal
- 1 cup all-purpose flour
- 1 tablespoon sugar
- 2 teaspoons baking powder

- ½ teaspoon baking soda
- ½ teaspoon salt
- 1 stick butter melted
- 1½ cups buttermilk
- 2 eggs
- 113g diced chiles

Directions:
1. Mix cornmeal with flour, sugar, baking powder, baking soda, salt, butter, milk, eggs and chiles in a bowl until smooth.
2. Spread this mixture in two greased 4-inch baking pans.
3. Place one pan in each air fryer basket.
4. Return the air fryer basket 1 to Zone 1, and basket 2 to Zone 2 of the Ninja Foodi 2-Basket Air Fryer.
5. Choose the "Air Fry" mode for Zone 1 at 330 degrees F and 15 minutes of cooking time.
6. Select the "MATCH COOK" option to copy the settings for Zone 2.
7. Initiate cooking by pressing the START/PAUSE BUTTON.
8. Slice and serve.

Nutrition Info:
- (Per serving) Calories 199 | Fat 11.1g |Sodium 297mg | Carbs 14.9g | Fiber 1g | Sugar 2.5g | Protein 9.9g

Quiche Breakfast Peppers

Servings: 4
Cooking Time: 15 Minutes
Ingredients:
- 4 eggs
- ½ tsp garlic powder
- 112g mozzarella cheese, shredded
- 125g ricotta cheese
- 2 bell peppers, cut in half & remove seeds
- 7½g baby spinach, chopped
- 22g parmesan cheese, grated
- ¼ tsp dried parsley

Directions:
1. In a bowl, whisk eggs, ricotta cheese, garlic powder, parsley, cheese, and spinach.
2. Pour the egg mixture into each bell pepper half and top with mozzarella cheese.
3. Insert a crisper plate in the Ninja Foodi air fryer baskets.
4. Place bell peppers in both the baskets.
5. Select zone 1 then select "air fry" mode and set the temperature to 355 degrees F for 15 minutes. Press "match" to match zone 2 settings to zone 1. Press "start/stop" to begin.

Nutrition Info:
- (Per serving) Calories 136 | Fat 7.6g |Sodium 125mg | Carbs 6.9g | Fiber 0.9g | Sugar 3.5g | Protein 10.8g

Lemon-cream Cheese Danishes
Cherry Danishes

Servings:4
Cooking Time: 15 Minutes
Ingredients:
- FOR THE CREAM CHEESE DANISHES
- 1 ounce (2 tablespoons) cream cheese, at room temperature
- 1 teaspoon granulated sugar
- ¼ teaspoon freshly squeezed lemon juice
- ⅛ teaspoon vanilla extract
- ½ sheet frozen puff pastry, thawed
- 2 tablespoons lemon curd
- 1 large egg yolk
- 1 tablespoon water
- FOR THE CHERRY DANISHES
- ½ sheet frozen puff pastry, thawed
- 2 tablespoons cherry preserves
- 1 teaspoon coarse sanding sugar

Directions:
1. To prep the cream cheese Danishes: In a small bowl, mix the cream cheese, granulated sugar, lemon juice, and vanilla.
2. Cut the puff pastry sheet into 2 squares. Cut a ½-inch-wide strip from each side of the pastry. Brush the edges of the pastry square with water, then layer the strips along the edges, pressing gently to adhere and form a border around the outside of the pastry.
3. Divide the cream cheese mixture between the two pastries, then top each with 1 tablespoon of lemon curd.
4. In a second small bowl, whisk together the egg yolk and water (this will be used for the cherry Danishes, too). Brush the exposed edges of the pastry with half the egg wash.
5. To prep the cherry Danishes: Cut the puff pastry sheet into 2 squares. Cut a ½-inch-wide strip from each side of the pastry. Brush the edges of the pastry square with water, then layer the strips along the edges, pressing gently to adhere and form a border around the outside of the pastry.
6. Spoon 1 tablespoon of cherry preserves into the center of each pastry.
7. Brush the exposed edges of the pastry with the remaining egg wash, then sprinkle with the sanding sugar.
8. To cook both Danishes: Install a crisper plate in each of the two baskets. Place the cream cheese Danishes in the Zone 1 basket and insert the basket in the unit. Place the cherry Danishes in the Zone 2 basket and insert the basket in the unit.
9. Select Zone 1, select AIR FRY, set the temperature to 330°F, and set the time to 15 minutes. Select MATCH COOK to match Zone 2 settings to Zone 1.
10. Press START/PAUSE to begin cooking.

11. When cooking is complete, transfer the Danishes to a wire rack to cool. Serve warm.
Nutrition Info:
- (Per serving) Calories: 415; Total fat: 24g; Saturated fat: 12g; Carbohydrates: 51g; Fiber: 1.5g; Protein: 7g; Sodium: 274mg

Sweet Potato Hash

Servings: 4
Cooking Time: 15 Minutes
Ingredients:
- 3 sweet potatoes, peel & cut into ½-inch pieces
- ½ tsp cinnamon
- 2 tbsp olive oil
- 1 bell pepper, cut into ½-inch pieces
- ½ tsp dried thyme
- ½ tsp nutmeg
- 1 medium onion, cut into ½-inch pieces
- Pepper
- Salt

Directions:
1. In a bowl, toss sweet potatoes with the remaining ingredients.
2. Insert a crisper plate in Ninja Foodi air fryer baskets.
3. Add potato mixture in both baskets.
4. Select zone 1 then select "air fry" mode and set the temperature to 355 degrees F for 15 minutes. Press "match" to match zone 2 settings to zone 1. Press "start/stop" to begin.

Nutrition Info:
- (Per serving) Calories 167 | Fat 7.3g |Sodium 94mg | Carbs 24.9g | Fiber 4.2g | Sugar 6.8g | Protein 2.2g

Sausage Hash And Baked Eggs

Servings:4
Cooking Time: 30 Minutes
Ingredients:
- FOR THE HASH
- 2 yellow potatoes (about 1 pound), cut into ½-inch pieces
- 4 garlic cloves, minced
- 1 teaspoon kosher salt
- ¼ teaspoon freshly ground black pepper
- 2 tablespoons olive oil
- ½ pound pork breakfast sausage meat
- 1 small yellow onion, diced
- 1 red bell pepper, diced
- 1 teaspoon Italian seasoning
- FOR THE EGGS
- Nonstick cooking spray
- 4 large eggs
- 4 tablespoons water

Directions:
1. To prep the hash: In a large bowl, combine the potatoes, garlic, salt, black pepper, and olive oil and toss to coat. Crumble in the sausage and mix until combined.
2. To prep the eggs: Mist 4 silicone muffin cups with cooking spray. Crack 1 egg into each muffin cup. Top each egg with 1 tablespoon of water.
3. To cook the hash and eggs: Install a crisper plate in the Zone 1 basket. Place the sausage and potato mixture in the Zone 1 basket and insert the basket in the unit. Place the egg cups in the Zone 2 basket and insert the basket in the unit.
4. Select Zone 1, select AIR FRY, set the temperature to 400°F, and set the time to 30 minutes.
5. Select Zone 2, select BAKE, set the temperature to 325°F, and set the time to 12 minutes. Select SMART FINISH.
6. Press START/PAUSE to begin cooking.
7. When the Zone 1 timer reads 20 minutes, press START/PAUSE. Remove the basket and add the onion, bell pepper, and Italian seasoning to the hash. Mix until combined, breaking up any large pieces of sausage. Reinsert the basket and press START/PAUSE to resume cooking.
8. When cooking is complete, serve the hash topped with an egg.

Nutrition Info:
- (Per serving) Calories: 400; Total fat: 23g; Saturated fat: 5.5g; Carbohydrates: 31g; Fiber: 2g; Protein: 19g; Sodium: 750mg

Banana Muffins

Servings: 10
Cooking Time: 15 Minutes
Ingredients:
- 2 very ripe bananas
- ⅓ cup olive oil
- 1 egg
- ½ cup brown sugar
- 1 teaspoon vanilla extract
- 1 teaspoon cinnamon
- ¾ cup self-rising flour

Directions:
1. In a large mixing bowl, mash the bananas, then add the egg, brown sugar, olive oil, and vanilla. To blend, stir everything together thoroughly.
2. Fold in the flour and cinnamon until everything is just blended.
3. Fill muffin molds evenly with the mixture (silicone or paper).
4. Install a crisper plate in both drawers. Place the muffin molds in a single layer in each drawer. Insert the drawers into the unit.
5. Select zone 1, select AIR FRY, set temperature to 360 degrees F/ 180 degrees C, and set time to 15 minutes. Select MATCH to match zone 2 settings to zone 1. Select START/STOP to begin.

6. Once the timer has finished, remove the muffins from the drawers.
7. Serve and enjoy!
Nutrition Info:
- (Per serving) Calories 148 | Fat 7.3g | Sodium 9mg | Carbs 19.8g | Fiber 1g | Sugar 10g | Protein 1.8g

Breakfast Stuffed Peppers

Servings: 4
Cooking Time: 13 Minutes
Ingredients:
- 2 capsicums, halved, seeds removed
- 4 eggs
- 1 teaspoon olive oil
- 1 pinch salt and pepper
- 1 pinch sriracha flakes

Directions:
1. Cut each capsicum in half and place two halves in each air fryer basket.
2. Crack one egg into each capsicum and top it with black pepper, salt, sriracha flakes and olive oil.
3. Return the air fryer basket 1 to Zone 1, and basket 2 to Zone 2 of the Ninja Foodi 2-Basket Air Fryer.
4. Choose the "Air Fry" mode for Zone 1 at 390 degrees F and 13 minutes of cooking time.
5. Select the "MATCH COOK" option to copy the settings for Zone 2.
6. Initiate cooking by pressing the START/PAUSE BUTTON.
7. Serve warm.

Nutrition Info:
- (Per serving) Calories 237 | Fat 19g |Sodium 518mg | Carbs 7g | Fiber 1.5g | Sugar 3.4g | Protein 12g

Sweet Potatoes Hash

Servings: 2
Cooking Time: 25
Ingredients:
- 450 grams sweet potatoes
- 1/2 white onion, diced
- 3 tablespoons of olive oil
- 1 teaspoon smoked paprika
- 1/4 teaspoon cumin
- 1/3 teaspoon of ground turmeric
- 1/4 teaspoon of garlic salt
- 1 cup guacamole

Directions:
1. Peel and cut the potatoes into cubes.
2. Now, transfer the potatoes to a bowl and add oil, white onions, cumin, paprika, turmeric, and garlic salt.
3. Put this mixture between both the baskets of the Ninja Foodie 2-Basket Air Fryer.
4. Set it to AIR FRY mode for 10 minutes at 390 degrees F.
5. Then take out the baskets and shake them well.
6. Then again set time to 15 minutes at 390 degrees F.
7. Once done, serve it with guacamole.

Nutrition Info:
- (Per serving) Calories691 | Fat 49.7g| Sodium 596mg | Carbs 64g | Fiber15g | Sugar 19g | Protein 8.1g

Blueberry Coffee Cake And Maple Sausage Patties

Servings:6
Cooking Time: 25 Minutes
Ingredients:
- FOR THE COFFEE CAKE
- 6 tablespoons unsalted butter, at room temperature, divided
- ⅓ cup granulated sugar
- 1 large egg
- 1 teaspoon vanilla extract
- ¼ cup whole milk
- 1½ cups all-purpose flour, divided
- 1 teaspoon baking powder
- ¼ teaspoon salt
- 1 cup blueberries
- ¼ cup packed light brown sugar
- ½ teaspoon ground cinnamon
- FOR THE SAUSAGE PATTIES
- ½ pound ground pork
- 2 tablespoons maple syrup
- ½ teaspoon dried sage
- ½ teaspoon dried thyme
- 1½ teaspoons kosher salt
- ½ teaspoon crushed fennel seeds
- ½ teaspoon red pepper flakes (optional)
- ¼ teaspoon freshly ground black pepper

Directions:
1. To prep the coffee cake: In a large bowl, cream together 4 tablespoons of butter with the granulated sugar. Beat in the egg, vanilla, and milk.
2. Stir in 1 cup of flour, along with the baking soda and salt, to form a thick batter. Fold in the blueberries.
3. In a second bowl, mix the remaining 2 tablespoons of butter, remaining ½ cup of flour, the brown sugar, and cinnamon to form a dry crumbly mixture.
4. To prep the sausage patties: In a large bowl, mix the pork, maple syrup, sage, thyme, salt, fennel seeds, red pepper flakes (if using), and black pepper until just combined.
5. Divide the mixture into 6 equal patties about ½ inch thick.
6. To cook the coffee cake and sausage patties: Spread the cake batter into the Zone 1 basket, top with the crumble mixture, and insert the basket in the unit. Install a crisper plate in the Zone 2 basket, add the sausage patties in a single layer, and insert the basket in the unit.
7. Select Zone 1, select BAKE, set the temperature to 350°F, and set the time to 25 minutes.

8. Select Zone 2, select AIR FRY, set the temperature to 375°F, and set the time to 12 minutes. Select SMART FINISH.
9. Press START/PAUSE to begin cooking.
10. When the Zone 2 timer reads 6 minutes, press START/PAUSE. Remove the basket and use silicone-tipped tongs to flip the sausage patties. Reinsert the basket and press START/PAUSE to resume cooking.
11. When cooking is complete, let the coffee cake cool for at least 5 minutes, then cut into 6 slices. Serve warm or at room temperature with the sausage patties.

Nutrition Info:
- (Per serving) Calories: 395; Total fat: 15g; Saturated fat: 8g; Carbohydrates: 53g; Fiber: 1.5g; Protein: 14g; Sodium: 187mg

Breakfast Frittata

Servings: 4
Cooking Time: 12 Minutes

Ingredients:
- 4 eggs
- 4 tablespoons milk
- 35g cheddar cheese grated
- 50g feta crumbled
- 1 tomato, deseeded and chopped
- 15g spinach chopped
- 1 tablespoon fresh herbs, chopped
- 2 spring onion chopped
- Salt and black pepper, to taste
- ½ teaspoon olive oil

Directions:
1. Beat eggs with milk in a bowl and stir in the rest of the ingredients.
2. Grease two small-sized springform pans and line them with parchment paper.
3. Divide the egg mixture into the pans and place one in each air fryer basket.
4. Return the air fryer basket 1 to Zone 1, and basket 2 to Zone 2 of the Ninja Foodi 2-Basket Air Fryer.
5. Choose the "Air Fry" mode for Zone 1 at 350 degrees F and 12 minutes of cooking time.
6. Select the "MATCH COOK" option to copy the settings for Zone 2.
7. Initiate cooking by pressing the START/PAUSE BUTTON.
8. Serve warm.

Nutrition Info:
- (Per serving) Calories 273 | Fat 22g |Sodium 517mg | Carbs 3.3g | Fiber 0.2g | Sugar 1.4g | Protein 16.1g

Air Fried Sausage

Servings: 4
Cooking Time: 13 Minutes.

Ingredients:
- 4 sausage links, raw and uncooked

Directions:
1. Divide the sausages in the two crisper plates.
2. Return the crisper plate to the Ninja Foodi Dual Zone Air Fryer.
3. Choose the Air Fry mode for Zone 1 and set the temperature to 390 degrees F and set the time to 13 minutes.
4. Select the "MATCH" button to copy the settings for Zone 2.
5. Initiate cooking by pressing the START/STOP button.
6. Serve warm and fresh.

Nutrition Info:
- (Per serving) Calories 267 | Fat 12g |Sodium 165mg | Carbs 39g | Fiber 1.4g | Sugar 22g | Protein 3.3g

Perfect Cinnamon Toast

Servings: 6
Cooking Time: 10 Minutes

Ingredients:
- 12 slices whole-wheat bread
- 1 stick butter, room temperature
- ½ cup white sugar
- 1½ teaspoons ground cinnamon
- 1½ teaspoons pure vanilla extract
- 1 pinch kosher salt
- 2 pinches freshly ground black pepper (optional)

Directions:
1. Mash the softened butter with a fork or the back of a spoon in a bowl. Add the sugar, cinnamon, vanilla, and salt. Stir until everything is well combined.
2. Spread one-sixth of the mixture onto each slice of bread, making sure to cover the entire surface.
3. Install a crisper plate in both drawers. Place half the bread sliced in the zone 1 drawer and half in the zone 2 drawer, then insert the drawers into the unit.
4. Select zone 1, select AIR FRY, set temperature to 400 degrees F/ 200 degrees C, and set time to 5 minutes. Select MATCH to match zone 2 settings to zone 1. Press theSTART/STOP button to begin cooking
5. When cooking is complete, remove the slices and cut them diagonally.
6. Serve immediately.

Nutrition Info:
- (Per serving) Calories 322 | Fat 16.5g | Sodium 249mg | Carbs 39.3g | Fiber 4.2g | Sugar 18.2g | Protein 8.2g

Pepper Egg Cups

Servings: 4
Cooking Time: 18 Minutes.

Ingredients:
- 2 halved bell pepper, seeds removed
- 4 eggs
- 1 teaspoon olive oil
- 1 pinch salt and black pepper
- 1 pinch sriracha flakes

Directions:
1. Slice the bell peppers in half, lengthwise, and remove their seeds and the inner portion to get a cup-like shape.
2. Rub olive oil on the edges of the bell peppers.
3. Place them in the two crisper plates with their cut side up and crack 1 egg in each half of bell pepper.
4. Drizzle salt, black pepper, and sriracha flakes on top of the eggs.
5. Return the crisper plates to the Ninja Foodi Dual Zone Air Fryer.
6. Choose the Air Fry mode for Zone 1 and set the temperature to 390 degrees F and the time to 18 minutes.
7. Select the "MATCH" button to copy the settings for Zone 2.
8. Initiate cooking by pressing the START/STOP button.
9. Serve warm and fresh.

Nutrition Info:
- (Per serving) Calories 183 | Fat 15g |Sodium 402mg | Carbs 2.5g | Fiber 0.4g | Sugar 1.1g | Protein 10g

Buttermilk Biscuits With Roasted Stone Fruit Compote

Servings:4
Cooking Time: 20 Minutes

Ingredients:
- FOR THE BISCUITS
- 1⅓ cups all-purpose flour
- 2 teaspoons sugar
- 2 teaspoons baking powder
- ½ teaspoon baking soda
- ½ teaspoon kosher salt
- 4 tablespoons (½ stick) very cold unsalted butter
- ½ cup plus 1 tablespoon low-fat buttermilk
- FOR THE FRUIT COMPOTE
- 2 peaches, peeled and diced
- 2 plums, peeled and diced
- ¼ cup water
- 2 teaspoons honey
- ⅛ teaspoon ground ginger (optional)

Directions:
1. To prep the biscuits: In a small bowl, combine the flour, sugar, baking powder, baking soda, and salt. Using the large holes on a box grater, grate in the butter. Stir in the buttermilk to form a thick dough.
2. Place the dough on a lightly floured surface and gently pat it into a ½-inch-thick disc. Fold the dough in half, then rotate the whole thing 90 degrees, pat into a ½-inch thick disc and fold again. Repeat until you have folded the dough four times.
3. Pat the dough out a final time into a ½-inch-thick disc and use a 3-inch biscuit cutter to cut 4 biscuits from the dough (discard the scraps).
4. To prep the fruit compote: In a large bowl, stir together the peaches, plums, water, honey, and ginger (if using).
5. To cook the biscuits and compote: Install a crisper plate in the Zone 1 basket, place the biscuits in the basket, and insert the basket in the unit. Place the fruit in the Zone 2 basket and insert the basket in the unit.
6. Select Zone 1, select AIR FRY, set the temperature to 400°F, and set the time to 10 minutes.
7. Select Zone 2, select ROAST, set the temperature to 350°F, and set the time to 20 minutes. Select SMART FINISH.
8. Press START/PAUSE to begin cooking.
9. When the Zone 2 timer reads 10 minutes, press START/PAUSE. Remove the basket and stir the compote. Reinsert the basket and press START/PAUSE to resume cooking.
10. When cooking is complete, the biscuits will be golden brown and crisp on top and the fruit will be soft. Transfer the biscuits to a plate to cool. Lightly mash the fruit to form a thick, jammy sauce.
11. Split the biscuits in half horizontally and serve topped with fruit compote.

Nutrition Info:
- (Per serving) Calories: 332; Total fat: 12g; Saturated fat: 7.5g; Carbohydrates: 50g; Fiber: 2.5g; Protein: 6g; Sodium: 350mg

Egg White Muffins

Servings: 8
Cooking Time: 10 Minutes

Ingredients:
- 4 slices center-cut bacon, cut into strips
- 4 ounces baby bella mushrooms, roughly chopped
- 2 ounces sun-dried tomatoes
- 2 tablespoon sliced black olives
- 2 tablespoons grated or shredded parmesan
- 2 tablespoons shredded mozzarella
- ¼ teaspoon black pepper
- ¾ cup liquid egg whites
- 2 tablespoons liquid egg whites

Directions:
1. Heat a saucepan with a little oil, add the bacon and mushrooms and cook until fully cooked and crispy, about 6–8 minutes.
2. While the bacon and mushrooms cook, mix the ¾ cup liquid egg whites, sun-dried tomato, olives, parmesan, mozzarella, and black pepper together in a large bowl.
3. Add the cooked bacon and mushrooms to the tomato and olive mixture, stirring everything together.
4. Spoon the mixture into muffin molds, followed by 2 tablespoons of egg whites over the top.
5. Place half the muffins mold in zone 1 and half in zone 2, then insert the drawers into the unit.

6. Select zone 1, select AIR FRY, set temperature to 390 degrees F/ 200 degrees C, and set time to 22 minutes.
7. Select MATCH to match zone 2 settings to zone 1. Press the START/STOP button to begin cooking.
8. When cooking is complete, remove the molds and enjoy!

Nutrition Info:
- (Per serving) Calories 104 | Fat 5.6g | Sodium 269mg | Carbs 3.5g | Fiber 0.8g | Sugar 0.3g | Protein 10.3g

Sweet Potato Sausage Hash

Servings: 4
Cooking Time: 20 Minutes

Ingredients:
- 1½ pounds sweet potato, peeled and diced into ½-inch pieces
- 1 tablespoon minced garlic
- 1 teaspoon kosher salt plus more, as desired
- Ground black pepper, as desired
- 2 tablespoons canola oil
- 1 tablespoon dried sage
- 1-pound uncooked mild ground breakfast sausage
- ½ large onion, peeled and diced
- ½ teaspoon ground cinnamon
- 1 teaspoon chili powder
- 4 large eggs, poached or fried (optional)

Directions:
1. Toss the sweet potatoes with the garlic, salt, pepper, and canola oil in a mixing bowl.
2. Install the crisper plate in the zone 1 drawer, fill it with the sweet potato mixture, and insert the drawer in the unit.
3. Place the ground sausage in the zone 2 drawer (without the crisper plate) and place it in the unit.
4. Select zone 1, then AIR FRY, and set the temperature to 400 degrees F/ 200 degrees C with a 30-minute timer.
5. Select zone 2, then ROAST, then set the temperature to 400 degrees F/ 200 degrees C with a 20-minute timer. SYNC is the option to choose. To begin cooking, press the START/STOP button.
6. When the zone 1 and zone 2 times have reached 10 minutes, press START/STOP and remove the drawers from the unit. Shake each for 10 seconds.
7. Half of the sage should be added to the zone 1 drawer.
8. Add the onion to the zone 2 drawer and mix to incorporate. To continue cooking, press START/STOP and reinsert the drawers.
9. Remove both drawers from the unit once the cooking is finished and add the potatoes to the sausage mixture. Mix in the cinnamon, sage, chili powder, and salt until thoroughly combined.
10. When the hash is done, stir it and serve it right away with a poached or fried egg on top, if desired.

Nutrition Info:
- (Per serving) Calories 491 | Fat 19.5g | Sodium 736mg | Carbs 51g | Fiber 8g | Sugar 2g | Protein 26.3

Egg With Baby Spinach

Servings: 4
Cooking Time: 12

Ingredients:
- Nonstick spray, for greasing ramekins
- 2 tablespoons olive oil
- 6 ounces baby spinach
- 2 garlic cloves, minced
- 1/3 teaspoon kosher salt
- 6-8 large eggs
- ½ cup half and half
- Salt and black pepper, to taste
- 8 Sourdough bread slices, toasted

Directions:
1. Grease 4 ramekins with oil spray and set aside for further use.
2. Take a skillet and heat oil in it.
3. Then cook spinach for 2 minutes and add garlic and salt black pepper.
4. Let it simmer for 2 more minutes.
5. Once the spinach is wilted, transfer it to a plate.
6. Whisk an egg into a small bowl.
7. Add in the spinach.
8. Whisk it well and then pour half and half
9. Divide this mixture between 4 ramekins and remember not to overfill it to the top, leave a little space on top.
10. Put the ramekins in zone 1 and zone 2 baskets of the Ninja Foodie 2-Basket Air Fryer.
11. Press start and set zone 1 to AIR fry it at 350 degrees F for 8-12 minutes.
12. Press the MATCH button for zone 2.
13. Once it's cooked and eggs are done, serve with sourdough bread slices.

Nutrition Info:
- (Per serving) Calories 404| Fat 19.6g| Sodium 761mg | Carbs 40.1g| Fiber 2.5g| Sugar 2.5g | Protein 19.2g

Morning Egg Rolls

Servings: 6
Cooking Time: 13 Minutes.

Ingredients:
- 2 eggs
- 2 tablespoons milk
- Salt, to taste
- Black pepper, to taste
- ½ cup shredded cheddar cheese
- 2 sausage patties
- 6 egg roll wrappers

- 1 tablespoon olive oil
- 1 cup water

Directions:
1. Grease a small skillet with some olive oil and place it over medium heat.
2. Add sausage patties and cook them until brown.
3. Chop the cooked patties into small pieces. Beat eggs with salt, black pepper, and milk in a mixing bowl.
4. Grease the same skillet with 1 teaspoon of olive oil and pour the egg mixture into it.
5. Stir cook to make scrambled eggs.
6. Add sausage, mix well and remove the skillet from the heat.
7. Spread an egg roll wrapper on the working surface in a diamond shape position.
8. Add a tablespoon of cheese at the bottom third of the roll wrapper.
9. Top the cheese with egg mixture and wet the edges of the wrapper with water.
10. Fold the two corners of the wrapper and roll it, then seal the edges.
11. Repeat the same steps and divide the rolls in the two crisper plates.
12. Return the crisper plates to the Ninja Foodi Dual Zone Air Fryer.
13. Choose the Air Fry mode for Zone 1 and set the temperature to 375 degrees F and the time to 13 minutes.
14. Select the "MATCH" button to copy the settings for Zone 2.
15. Initiate cooking by pressing the START/STOP button.
16. Flip the rolls after 8 minutes and continue cooking for another 5 minutes.
17. Serve warm and fresh.

Nutrition Info:
- (Per serving) Calories 282 | Fat 15g |Sodium 526mg | Carbs 20g | Fiber 0.6g | Sugar 3.3g | Protein 16g

Sausage & Butternut Squash

Servings: 2
Cooking Time: 20 Minutes
Ingredients:
- 450g butternut squash, diced
- 70g kielbasa, diced
- ¼ onion, diced
- ¼ tsp garlic powder
- ½ tbsp olive oil
- Pepper
- Salt

Directions:
1. In a bowl, toss butternut squash with garlic powder, oil, onion, kielbasa, pepper, and salt.
2. Insert a crisper plate in the Ninja Foodi air fryer baskets.
3. Add sausage and butternut squash mixture in both baskets.
4. Select zone 1, then select "air fry" mode and set the temperature to 375 degrees F for 20 minutes. Press "match" to match zone 2 settings to zone 1. Press "start/stop" to begin. Stir halfway through.

Nutrition Info:
- (Per serving) Calories 68 | Fat 3.6g |Sodium 81mg | Carbs 9.7g | Fiber 1.7g | Sugar 2.2g | Protein 0.9g

Cheesy Baked Eggs

Servings: 4
Cooking Time: 16 Minutes
Ingredients:
- 4 large eggs
- 57g smoked gouda, shredded
- Everything bagel seasoning, to taste
- Salt and pepper to taste

Directions:
1. Crack one egg in each ramekin.
2. Top the egg with bagel seasoning, black pepper, salt and gouda.
3. Place 2 ramekins in each air fryer basket.
4. Return the air fryer basket 1 to Zone 1, and basket 2 to Zone 2 of the Ninja Foodi 2-Basket Air Fryer.
5. Choose the "Air Fry" mode for Zone 1 and set the temperature to 400 degrees F and 16 minutes of cooking time.
6. Select the "MATCH COOK" option to copy the settings for Zone 2.
7. Initiate cooking by pressing the START/PAUSE BUTTON.
8. Serve warm.

Nutrition Info:
- (Per serving) Calories 190 | Fat 18g |Sodium 150mg | Carbs 0.6g | Fiber 0.4g | Sugar 0.4g | Protein 7.2g

Hash Browns

Servings: 4
Cooking Time: 5 Minutes
Ingredients:
- 4 frozen hash browns patties
- Cooking oil spray of choice

Directions:
1. Install a crisper plate in both drawers. Place half the hash browns in zone 1 and half in zone 2, then insert the drawers into the unit. Spray the hash browns with some cooking oil.
2. Select zone 1, select AIR FRY, set temperature to 390 degrees F/ 200 degrees C, and set time to 5 minutes.
3. Select MATCH to match zone 2 settings to zone 1. Press the START/STOP button to begin cooking.
4. When cooking is complete, remove the hash browns and serve.

Nutrition Info:
- (Per serving) Calories 130 | Fat 7g | Sodium 300mg | Carbs 15g | Fiber 2g | Sugar 0g | Protein 1g

Bagels

Servings: 8
Cooking Time: 15 Minutes
Ingredients:
- 2 cups self-rising flour
- 2 cups non-fat plain Greek yogurt
- 2 beaten eggs for egg wash (optional)
- ½ cup sesame seeds (optional)

Directions:
1. In a medium mixing bowl, combine the self-rising flour and Greek yogurt using a wooden spoon.
2. Knead the dough for about 5 minutes on a lightly floured board.
3. Divide the dough into four equal pieces and roll each into a thin rope, securing the ends to form a bagel shape.
4. Install a crisper plate in both drawers. Place 4 bagels in a single layer in each drawer. Insert the drawers into the unit.
5. Select zone 1, select AIR FRY, set temperature to 360 degrees F/ 180 degrees C, and set time to 15 minutes. Select MATCH to match zone 2 settings to zone 1. Select START/STOP to begin.
6. Once the timer has finished, remove the bagels from the units.
7. Serve and enjoy!

Nutrition Info:
- (Per serving) Calories 202 | Fat 4.5g | Sodium 55mg | Carbs 31.3g | Fiber 2.7g | Sugar 4.7g | Protein 8.7g

Egg And Avocado In The Ninja Foodi

Servings: 2
Cooking Time: 12
Ingredients:
- 2 Avocados, pitted and cut in half
- Garlic salt, to taste
- Cooking for greasing
- 4 eggs
- ¼ teaspoon of Paprika powder, for sprinkling
- 1/3 cup parmesan cheese, crumbled
- 6 bacon strips, raw

Directions:
1. First cut the avocado in half and pit it.
2. Now scoop out the flesh from the avocado and keep intact some of it
3. Crack one egg in each hole of avocado and sprinkle paprika and garlic salt
4. Top it with cheese at the end.
5. Now put it into tin foils and then put it in the air fryer zone basket 1
6. Put bacon strips in zone 2 basket.
7. Now for zone 1, set it to AIR FRY mode at 350 degrees F for 10 minutes
8. And for zone 2, set it 400 degrees for 12 minutes AIR FRY mode.
9. Press the Smart finish button and press start, it will finish both at the same time.
10. Once done, serve and enjoy.

Nutrition Info:
- (Per serving) Calories 609 | Fat 53.2g | Sodium 335mg | Carbs 18.1g | Fiber 13.5g | Sugar 1.7g | Protein 21.3g

Banana And Raisins Muffins

Servings: 2
Cooking Time: 16
Ingredients:
- Salt, pinch
- 2 eggs, whisked
- 1/3 cup butter, melted
- 4 tablespoons of almond milk
- ¼ teaspoon of vanilla extract
- ½ teaspoon of baking powder
- 1-1/2 cup all-purpose flour
- 1 cup mashed bananas
- 2 tablespoons of raisins

Directions:
1. Take about 4 large (one-cup sized) ramekins and layer them with muffin papers.
2. Crack eggs in a large bowl, and whisk it all well and start adding vanilla extract, almond milk, baking powder, and melted butter
3. Whisk the ingredients very well.
4. Take a separate bowl and add the all-purpose flour, and salt.
5. Now, combine the add dry ingredients with the wet ingredients.
6. Now, pour mashed bananas and raisins into this batter
7. Mix it well to make a batter for the muffins.
8. Now pour the batter into four ramekins and divided the ramekins in the air fryer zones.
9. Set the timer for zone 1 to 16 minutes at 350 degrees F.
10. Select the MATCH button for the zone 2 basket.
11. Check if not done, and let it AIR FRY for one more minute.
12. Once it is done, serve.

Nutrition Info:
- (Per serving) Calories 727 | Fat 43.1g | Sodium 366 mg | Carbs 74.4g | Fiber 4.7g | Sugar 16.1g | Protein 14.1g

Breakfast Sausage Omelet

Servings: 2
Cooking Time: 8
Ingredients:
- ¼ pound breakfast sausage, cooked and crumbled
- 4 eggs, beaten
- ½ cup pepper Jack cheese blend
- 2 tablespoons green bell pepper, sliced
- 1 green onion, chopped
- 1 pinch cayenne pepper
- Cooking spray

Directions:
1. Take a bowl and whisk eggs in it along with crumbled sausage, pepper Jack cheese, green onions, red bell pepper, and cayenne pepper.
2. Mix it all well.
3. Take two cake pans that fit inside the air fryer and grease it with oil spray.
4. Divide the omelet mixture between cake pans.
5. Put the cake pans inside both of the Ninja Foodie 2-Basket Air Fryer baskets.
6. Turn on the BAKE function of the zone 1 basket and let it cook for 15-20 minutes at 310 degrees F.
7. Select MATCH button for zone 2 basket.
8. Once the cooking cycle completes, take out, and serve hot, as a delicious breakfast.

Nutrition Info:
- (Per serving) Calories 691| Fat52.4g | Sodium1122 mg | Carbs 13.3g | Fiber 1.8g| Sugar 7g | Protein 42g

Sausage Breakfast Casserole

Servings: 4
Cooking Time: 10 Minutes
Ingredients:
- 455g hash browns
- 455g ground breakfast sausage
- 1 green capsicum diced
- 1 red capsicum diced
- 1 yellow capsicum diced
- ¼ cup sweet onion diced
- 4 eggs

Directions:
1. Layer each air fryer basket with parchment paper.
2. Place the hash browns in both the baskets.
3. Spread sausage, onion and peppers over the hash brown.
4. Return the air fryer basket 1 to Zone 1, and basket 2 to Zone 2 of the Ninja Foodi 2-Basket Air Fryer.
5. Choose the "Air Fry" mode for Zone 1 at 355 degrees F temperature and 10 minutes of cooking time.
6. Select the "MATCH COOK" option to copy the settings for Zone 2.
7. Initiate cooking by pressing the START/PAUSE BUTTON.
8. Beat eggs in a bowl and pour over the air fried veggies.
9. Continue air frying for 10 minutes.
10. Garnish with salt and black pepper.
11. Serve warm.

Nutrition Info:
- (Per serving) Calories 267 | Fat 12g |Sodium 165mg | Carbs 39g | Fiber 1.4g | Sugar 22g | Protein 3.3g

Crispy Hash Browns

Servings: 4
Cooking Time: 13 Minutes.
Ingredients:
- 3 russet potatoes
- ¼ cup chopped green peppers
- ¼ cup chopped red peppers
- ¼ cup chopped onions
- 2 garlic cloves chopped
- 1 teaspoon paprika
- Salt and black pepper, to taste
- 2 teaspoons olive oil

Directions:
1. Peel and grate all the potatoes with the help of a cheese grater.
2. Add potato shreds to a bowl filled with cold water and leave it soaked for 25 minutes.
3. Drain the water and place the potato shreds on a plate lined with a paper towel.
4. Transfer the shreds to a dry bowl and add olive oil, paprika, garlic, and black pepper.
5. Make four flat patties out of the potato mixture and place two into each of the crisper plate.
6. Return the crisper plate to the Ninja Foodi Dual Zone Air Fryer.
7. Choose the Air Fry mode for Zone 1 and set the temperature to 390 degrees F and set the time to 13 minutes.
8. Select the "MATCH" button to copy the settings for Zone 2.
9. Initiate cooking by pressing the START/STOP button.
10. Flip the potato hash browns once cooked halfway through, then resume cooking.
11. Once done, serve warm.

Nutrition Info:
- (Per serving) Calories 190 | Fat 18g |Sodium 150mg | Carbs 0.6g | Fiber 0.4g | Sugar 0.4g | Protein 7.2g

Turkey Ham Muffins

Servings: 16
Cooking Time: 10 Minutes
Ingredients:
- 1 egg
- 340g all-purpose flour
- 85g turkey ham, chopped
- 2 tbsp mix herbs, chopped

- 235g cheddar cheese, shredded
- 1 onion, chopped
- 2 tsp baking powder
- 2 tbsp butter, melted
- 237ml milk
- Pepper
- Salt

Directions:
1. In a large bowl, mix flour and baking powder.
2. Add egg, butter, and milk and mix until well combined.
3. Add herbs, cheese, onion, and turkey ham and mix well.
4. Insert a crisper plate in the Ninja Foodi air fryer baskets.
5. Pour the batter into the silicone muffin moulds.
6. Place muffin moulds in both baskets.
7. Select zone 1, then select "air fry" mode and set the temperature to 355 degrees F for 10 minutes. Press "match" to match zone 2 settings to zone 1. Press "start/stop" to begin.

Nutrition Info:
- (Per serving) Calories 140 | Fat 4.8g |Sodium 126mg | Carbs 18.2g | Fiber 0.7g | Sugar 1.2g | Protein 5.8g

Brussels Sprouts Potato Hash

Servings: 4
Cooking Time: 10 Minutes
Ingredients.
- 455g Brussels sprouts
- 1 small to medium red onion
- 227g baby red potatoes
- 2 tablespoons avocado oil
- ½ teaspoon salt
- ½ teaspoon black pepper

Directions:
1. Peel and boil potatoes in salted water for 15 minutes until soft.
2. Drain and allow them to cool down then dice.
3. Shred Brussels sprouts and toss them with potatoes and the rest of the ingredients.
4. Divide this veggies hash mixture in both of the air fryer baskets.
5. Return the air fryer basket 1 to Zone 1, and basket 2 to Zone 2 of the Ninja Foodi 2-Basket Air Fryer.
6. Choose the "Air Fry" mode for Zone 1 with 375 degrees F temperature and 10 minutes of cooking time.
7. Select the "MATCH COOK" option to copy the settings for Zone 2.
8. Initiate cooking by pressing the START/PAUSE BUTTON.
9. Shake the veggies once cooked halfway through.
10. Serve warm.

Nutrition Info:
- (Per serving) Calories 305 | Fat 25g |Sodium 532mg | Carbs 2.3g | Fiber 0.4g | Sugar 2g | Protein 18.3g

Glazed Apple Fritters Glazed Peach Fritters

Servings:4
Cooking Time: 12 Minutes
Ingredients:
- FOR THE FRITTERS
- ¾ cup all-purpose flour
- 2 tablespoons granulated sugar
- 1 teaspoon baking powder
- ½ teaspoon kosher salt
- ½ teaspoon ground cinnamon
- ⅓ cup whole milk
- 2 tablespoons cold unsalted butter, grated
- 1 large egg
- 1 teaspoon fresh lemon juice
- 1 apple, peeled and diced
- 1 peach, peeled and diced
- FOR THE GLAZE
- ½ cup powdered sugar
- 1 tablespoon whole milk
- ½ teaspoon vanilla extract
- ½ teaspoon ground cinnamon
- Pinch salt

Directions:
1. To prep the fritters: In a large bowl, combine the flour, granulated sugar, baking powder, salt, and cinnamon. Stir in the milk, butter, egg, and lemon juice to form a thick batter.
2. Transfer half of the batter to a second bowl. Fold the apples into one bowl and the peaches into the other.
3. To prep the glaze: In a small bowl, whisk together the powdered sugar, milk, vanilla, cinnamon, and salt until smooth. Set aside.
4. To cook the fritters: Install a crisper plate in each of the two baskets. Drop two ¼-cup scoops of the apple fritter batter into the Zone 1 basket and insert the basket in the unit. Drop two ¼-cup scoops of the peach fritter batter into the Zone 2 basket and insert the basket in the unit.
5. Select Zone 1, select AIR FRY, set the temperature to 345°F, and set the time to 10 minutes.
6. Select Zone 2, select AIR FRY, set the temperature to 345°F, and set the time to 12 minutes. Select SMART FINISH.
7. Press START/PAUSE to begin cooking.
8. When cooking is complete, transfer the fritters to a wire rack and drizzle the glaze over them. Serve warm or at room temperature.

Nutrition Info:
- (Per serving) Calories: 298; Total fat: 8g; Saturated fat: 4.5g; Carbohydrates: 53g; Fiber: 3g; Protein: 5g; Sodium: 170mg

Vanilla Strawberry Doughnuts

Servings: 8
Cooking Time: 15 Minutes
Ingredients:
- 1 egg
- ½ cup strawberries, diced
- 80ml cup milk
- 1 tsp cinnamon
- 1 tsp baking soda
- 136g all-purpose flour
- 2 tsp vanilla
- 2 tbsp butter, melted
- 73g sugar
- ½ tsp salt

Directions:
1. In a bowl, mix flour, cinnamon, baking soda, sugar, and salt.
2. In a separate bowl, whisk egg, milk, butter, and vanilla.
3. Pour egg mixture into the flour mixture and mix until well combined.
4. Add strawberries and mix well.
5. Pour batter into the silicone doughnut moulds.
6. Insert a crisper plate in the Ninja Foodi air fryer baskets.
7. Place doughnut moulds in both baskets.
8. Select zone 1, then select "air fry" mode and set the temperature to 320 degrees F for 15 minutes. Press "match" to match zone 2 settings to zone 1. Press "start/stop" to begin.

Nutrition Info:
- (Per serving) Calories 133 | Fat 3.8g |Sodium 339mg | Carbs 21.9g | Fiber 0.8g | Sugar 9.5g | Protein 2.7g

Cinnamon Apple French Toast

Servings: 8
Cooking Time: 10 Minutes
Ingredients:
- 1 egg, lightly beaten
- 4 bread slices
- 1 tbsp cinnamon
- 15ml milk
- 23ml maple syrup
- 45 ml applesauce

Directions:
1. In a bowl, whisk egg, milk, cinnamon, applesauce, and maple syrup.
2. Insert a crisper plate in the Ninja Foodi air fryer baskets.
3. Dip each slice in egg mixture and place in both baskets.
4. Select zone 1 then select "air fry" mode and set the temperature to 355 degrees F for 10 minutes. Press "match" to match zone 2 settings to zone 1. Press "start/stop" to begin.

Nutrition Info:
- (Per serving) Calories 64 | Fat 1.5g |Sodium 79mg | Carbs 10.8g | Fiber 1.3g | Sugar 4.8g | Protein 2.3g

Breakfast Bacon

Servings: 4
Cooking Time: 14 Minutes.
Ingredients:
- ½ lb. bacon slices

Directions:
1. Spread half of the bacon slices in each of the crisper plate evenly in a single layer.
2. Return the crisper plate to the Ninja Foodi Dual Zone Air Fryer.
3. Choose the Air Fry mode for Zone 1 and set the temperature to 390 degrees F and the time to 14 minutes.
4. Select the "MATCH" button to copy the settings for Zone 2.
5. Initiate cooking by pressing the START/STOP button.
6. Flip the crispy bacon once cooked halfway through, then resume cooking.
7. Serve.

Nutrition Info:
- (Per serving) Calories 273 | Fat 22g |Sodium 517mg | Carbs 3.3g | Fiber 0.2g | Sugar 1.4g | Protein 16.1g

Snacks And Appetizers Recipes

Peppered Asparagus

Servings: 6
Cooking Time: 16 Minutes.
Ingredients:
- 1 bunch of asparagus, trimmed
- Avocado or Olive Oil
- Himalayan salt, to taste
- Black pepper, to taste

Directions:
1. Divide the asparagus in the two crisper plate.
2. Toss the asparagus with salt, black pepper, and oil.
3. Return the crisper plate to the Ninja Foodi Dual Zone Air Fryer.
4. Choose the Air Fry mode for Zone 1 and set the temperature to 390 degrees F and the time to 16 minutes.
5. Select the "MATCH" button to copy the settings for Zone 2.
6. Initiate cooking by pressing the START/STOP button.
7. Serve warm.

Nutrition Info:
- (Per serving) Calories 163 | Fat 11.5g |Sodium 918mg | Carbs 8.3g | Fiber 4.2g | Sugar 0.2g | Protein 7.4g

Cauliflower Gnocchi

Servings: 5
Cooking Time: 17 Minutes.
Ingredients:
- 1 bag frozen cauliflower gnocchi
- 1 ½ tablespoons olive oil
- 1 teaspoon garlic powder
- 3 tablespoons parmesan, grated
- ½ teaspoon dried basil
- Salt to taste
- Fresh chopped parsley for topping

Directions:
1. Toss gnocchi with olive oil, garlic powder, 1 tablespoon of parmesan, salt, and basil in a bowl.
2. Divide the gnocchi in the two crisper plate.
3. Return the crisper plate to the Ninja Foodi Dual Zone Air Fryer.
4. Choose the Air Fry mode for Zone 1 and set the temperature to 400 degrees F and the time to 10 minutes.
5. Select the "MATCH" button to copy the settings for Zone 2.
6. Initiate cooking by pressing the START/STOP button.
7. Toss the gnocchi once cooked halfway through, then resume cooking.
8. Drizzle the remaining parmesan on top of the gnocchi and cook again for 7 minutes.
9. Serve warm.

Nutrition Info:
- (Per serving) Calories 134 | Fat 5.9g |Sodium 343mg | Carbs 9.5g | Fiber 0.5g | Sugar 1.1g | Protein 10.4g

Bacon Wrapped Tater Tots

Servings: 8
Cooking Time: 14 Minutes
Ingredients:
- 8 bacon slices
- 3 tablespoons honey
- ½ tablespoon chipotle chile powder
- 16 frozen tater tots

Directions:
1. Cut the bacon slices in half and wrap each tater tot with a bacon slice.
2. Brush the bacon with honey and drizzle chipotle chile powder over them.
3. Insert a toothpick to seal the bacon.
4. Place the wrapped tots in the air fryer baskets.
5. Return the air fryer basket 1 to Zone 1, and basket 2 to Zone 2 of the Ninja Foodi 2-Basket Air Fryer.
6. Choose the "Air Fry" mode for Zone 1 at 350 degrees F and 14 minutes of cooking time.
7. Select the "MATCH COOK" option to copy the settings for Zone 2.
8. Initiate cooking by pressing the START/PAUSE BUTTON.
9. Serve warm.

Nutrition Info:
- (Per serving) Calories 100 | Fat 2g |Sodium 480mg | Carbs 4g | Fiber 2g | Sugar 0g | Protein 18g

Fried Halloumi Cheese

Servings: 6
Cooking Time: 12 Minutes.
Ingredients:
- 1 block of halloumi cheese, sliced
- 2 teaspoons olive oil

Directions:
1. Divide the halloumi cheese slices in the crisper plate.
2. Drizzle olive oil over the cheese slices.
3. Return the crisper plate to the Ninja Foodi Dual Zone Air Fryer.
4. Choose the Air Fry mode for Zone 1 and set the temperature to 360 degrees F and the time to 12 minutes.
5. Flip the cheese slices once cooked halfway through.
6. Serve.

Nutrition Info:
- (Per serving) Calories 186 | Fat 3g |Sodium 223mg | Carbs 31g | Fiber 8.7g | Sugar 5.5g | Protein 9.7g

Spicy Chicken Tenders

Servings: 2
Cooking Time: 12
Ingredients:
- 2 large eggs, whisked
- 2 tablespoons lemon juice
- Salt and black pepper
- 1 pound of chicken tenders
- 1 cup Panko breadcrumbs
- 1/2 cup Italian bread crumb
- 1 teaspoon smoked paprika
- 1/4 teaspoon garlic powder
- 1/4 teaspoon onion powder
- 1/2 cup fresh grated parmesan cheese

Directions:
1. Take a bowl and whisk eggs in it and set aside for further use.
2. In a large bowl add lemon juice, paprika, salt, black pepper, garlic powder, onion powder
3. In a separate bowl mix Panko breadcrumbs, Italian bread crumbs, and parmesan cheese.
4. Dip the chicken tender in the spice mixture and coat the entire tender well.
5. Let the tenders sit for 1 hour.
6. Then dip each chicken tender in egg and then in bread crumbs.
7. Line both the basket of the air fryer with parchment paper.
8. Divide the tenders between the baskets.
9. Set zone 1 basket to air fry mode at 350 degrees F for 12 minutes.
10. Select the MATCH button for the zone 2 basket.
11. Once it's done, serve.

Nutrition Info:
- (Per serving) Calories 836| Fat 36g| Sodium1307 mg | Carbs 31.3g | Fiber 2.5g| Sugar3.3 g | Protein 95.3g

Chicken Crescent Wraps

Servings: 6
Cooking Time: 12 Minutes.
Ingredients:
- 3 tablespoons chopped onion
- 3 garlic cloves, peeled and minced
- ¾ (8 ounces) package cream cheese
- 6 tablespoons butter
- 2 boneless chicken breasts, cubed, cooked
- 3 (10 ounces) cans refrigerated crescent roll dough

Directions:
1. Heat oil in a skillet and add onion and garlic to sauté until soft.
2. Add cooked chicken, sautéed veggies, butter, and cream cheese to a blender.
3. Blend well until smooth. Spread the crescent dough over a flat surface.
4. Slice the dough into 12 rectangles.
5. Spoon the chicken mixture at the center of each rectangle.
6. Roll the dough to wrap the mixture and form a ball.
7. Divide these balls into the two crisper plate.
8. Return the crisper plate to the Ninja Foodi Dual Zone Air Fryer.
9. Choose the Air Fry mode for Zone 1 and set the temperature to 390 degrees F and the time to 12 minutes.
10. Select the "MATCH" button to copy the settings for Zone 2.
11. Initiate cooking by pressing the START/STOP button.
12. Serve warm.

Nutrition Info:
- (Per serving) Calories 100 | Fat 2g |Sodium 480mg | Carbs 4g | Fiber 2g | Sugar 0g | Protein 18g

Fried Pickles

Servings: 4
Cooking Time: 15 Minutes
Ingredients:
- 2 cups sliced dill pickles
- 1 cup flour
- 1 tablespoon garlic powder
- 1 tablespoon Cajun spice
- ½ tablespoon cayenne pepper
- Olive Oil or cooking spray

Directions:
1. Mix together the flour and spices in a bowl.
2. Coat the sliced pickles with the flour mixture.
3. Place a crisper plate in each drawer. Put the pickles in a single layer in each drawer. Insert the drawers into the unit.
4. Select zone 1, then AIR FRY, then set the temperature to 400 degrees F/ 200 degrees C with a 15-minute timer. To match zone 2 settings to zone 1, choose MATCH. To begin, select START/STOP.

Nutrition Info:
- (Per serving) Calories 161 | Fat 4.1g | Sodium 975mg | Carbs 27.5g | Fiber 2.2g | Sugar 1.5g | Protein 4g

Cheddar Quiche

Servings: 2
Cooking Time: 12
Ingredients:
- 4 eggs, organic
- 1-1/4 cup heavy cream
- Salt, pinch
- ½ cup broccoli florets
- ½ cup cheddar cheese, shredded and for sprinkling

Directions:
1. Take a Pyrex pitcher and crack two eggs in it.
2. And fill it with heavy cream, about half the way up.

3. Add in the salt and then add in the broccoli and pour this into two quiche dishes, and top it with shredded cheddar cheese.
4. Now divide it between both zones of baskets.
5. For zone 1, set the time to 10-12 minutes at 325 degrees F.
6. Select the MATCH button for the zone 2 basket.
7. Once done, serve hot.

Nutrition Info:
- (Per serving) Calories 454| Fat40g | Sodium 406mg | Carbs 4.2g | Fiber 0.6g| Sugar1.3 g | Protein 20g

Crab Cakes

Servings: 4
Cooking Time: 10 Minutes
Ingredients:
- 227g lump crab meat
- 1 red capsicum, chopped
- 3 green onions, chopped
- 3 tablespoons mayonnaise
- 3 tablespoons breadcrumbs
- 2 teaspoons old bay seasoning
- 1 teaspoon lemon juice

Directions:
1. Mix crab meat with capsicum, onions and the rest of the ingredients in a food processor.
2. Make 4 inch crab cakes out of this mixture.
3. Divide the crab cakes into the Ninja Foodi 2 Baskets Air Fryer baskets.
4. Return the air fryer basket 1 to Zone 1, and basket 2 to Zone 2 of the Ninja Foodi 2-Basket Air Fryer.
5. Choose the "Air Fry" mode for Zone 1 at 370 degrees F and 10 minutes of cooking time.
6. Select the "MATCH COOK" option to copy the settings for Zone 2.
7. Initiate cooking by pressing the START/PAUSE BUTTON.
8. Flip the crab cakes once cooked halfway through.
9. Serve warm.

Nutrition Info:
- (Per serving) Calories 163 | Fat 11.5g |Sodium 918mg | Carbs 8.3g | Fiber 4.2g | Sugar 0.2g | Protein 7.4g

Beef Jerky Pineapple Jerky

Servings:8
Cooking Time: 6 To 12 Hours
Ingredients:
- FOR THE BEEF JERKY
- ½ cup reduced-sodium soy sauce
- ¼ cup pineapple juice
- 1 tablespoon dark brown sugar
- 1 tablespoon Worcestershire sauce
- ½ teaspoon smoked paprika
- ¼ teaspoon freshly ground black pepper
- ¼ teaspoon red pepper flakes
- 1 pound beef bottom round, trimmed of excess fat, cut into ¼-inch-thick slices
- FOR THE PINEAPPLE JERKY
- 1 pound pineapple, cut into ⅛-inch-thick rounds, pat dry
- 1 teaspoon chili powder (optional)

Directions:
1. To prep the beef jerky: In a large zip-top bag, combine the soy sauce, pineapple juice, brown sugar, Worcestershire sauce, smoked paprika, black pepper, and red pepper flakes.
2. Add the beef slices, seal the bag, and toss to coat the meat in the marinade. Refrigerate overnight or for at least 8 hours.
3. Remove the beef slices and discard the marinade. Using a paper towel, pat the slices dry to remove excess marinade.
4. To prep the pineapple jerky: Sprinkle the pineapple with chili powder (if using).
5. To dehydrate the jerky: Arrange half of the beef slices in a single layer in the Zone 1 basket, making sure they do not overlap. Place a crisper plate on top of the beef slices and arrange the remaining slices in a single layer on top of the crisper plate. Insert the basket in the unit.
6. Repeat this process with the pineapple in the Zone 2 basket and insert the basket in the unit.
7. Select Zone 1, select DEHYDRATE, set the temperature to 150°F, and set the time to 8 hours.
8. Select Zone 2, select DEHYDRATE, set the temperature to 135°F, and set the time to 12 hours.
9. Press START/PAUSE to begin cooking.
10. When the Zone 1 timer reads 2 hours, press START/PAUSE. Remove the basket and check the beef jerky for doneness. If necessary, reinsert the basket and press START/PAUSE to resume cooking.

Nutrition Info:
- (Per serving) Calories: 171; Total fat: 6.5g; Saturated fat: 2g; Carbohydrates: 2g; Fiber: 0g; Protein: 25g; Sodium: 369mg

Strawberries And Walnuts Muffins

Servings:2
Cooking Time:15
Ingredients:
- Salt, pinch
- 2 eggs, whisked
- 1/3 cup maple syrup
- 1/3 cup coconut oil
- 4 tablespoons of water
- 1 teaspoon of orange zest
- ¼ teaspoon of vanilla extract
- ½ teaspoon of baking powder
- 1 cup all-purpose flour
- 1 cup strawberries, finely chopped

- 1/3 cup walnuts, chopped and roasted

Directions:
1. Take one cup size of 4 ramekins that are oven safe.
2. Layer it with muffin paper.
3. In a bowl and add egg, maple syrup, oil, water, vanilla extract, and orange zest.
4. Whisk it all very well
5. In a separate bowl, mix flour, baking powder, and salt.
6. Now add dry ingredients slowly to wet ingredients.
7. Now pour this batter into ramekins and top it with strawberries and walnuts.
8. Now divide it between both zones and set the time for zone 1 basket to 15 minutes at 350 degrees F.
9. Select the MATCH button for the zone 2 basket.
10. Check if not done let it AIR FRY FOR one more minute.
11. Once done, serve.

Nutrition Info:
- (Per serving) Calories 897| Fat 53.9g | Sodium 148mg | Carbs 92g | Fiber 4.7g| Sugar35.6 g | Protein 17.5g

Parmesan French Fries

Servings: 6
Cooking Time: 20 Minutes.

Ingredients:
- 3 medium russet potatoes
- 2 tablespoons parmesan cheese
- 2 tablespoons fresh parsley, chopped
- 1 tablespoon olive oil
- Salt, to taste

Directions:
1. Wash the potatoes and pass them through the fries' cutter to get ¼-inch-thick fries.
2. Place the fries in a colander and drizzle salt on top.
3. Leave these fries for 10 minutes, then rinse.
4. Toss the potatoes with parmesan cheese, oil, salt, and parsley in a bowl.
5. Divide the potatoes into the two crisper plates.
6. Return the crisper plates to the Ninja Foodi Dual Zone Air Fryer.
7. Choose the Air Fry mode for Zone 1 and set the temperature to 360 degrees F and the time to 20 minutes.
8. Select the "MATCH" button to copy the settings for Zone 2.
9. Initiate cooking by pressing the START/STOP button.
10. Toss the chips once cooked halfway through, then resume cooking.
11. Serve warm.

Nutrition Info:
- (Per serving) Calories 307 | Fat 8.6g |Sodium 510mg | Carbs 22.2g | Fiber 1.4g | Sugar 13g | Protein 33.6g

Onion Rings

Servings: 4
Cooking Time: 7 Minutes

Ingredients:
- 170g onion, sliced into rings
- ½ cup breadcrumbs
- 2 eggs, beaten
- ½ cup flour
- Salt and black pepper to taste

Directions:
1. Mix flour, black pepper and salt in a bowl.
2. Dredge the onion rings through the flour mixture.
3. Dip them in the eggs and coat with the breadcrumbs.
4. Place the coated onion rings in the air fryer baskets.
5. Return the air fryer basket 1 to Zone 1, and basket 2 to Zone 2 of the Ninja Foodi 2-Basket Air Fryer.
6. Choose the "Air Fry" mode for Zone 1 at 350 degrees F and 7 minutes of cooking time.
7. Select the "MATCH COOK" option to copy the settings for Zone 2.
8. Initiate cooking by pressing the START/PAUSE BUTTON.
9. Shake the rings once cooked halfway through.
10. Serve warm.

Nutrition Info:
- (Per serving) Calories 185 | Fat 11g |Sodium 355mg | Carbs 21g | Fiber 5.8g | Sugar 3g | Protein 4.7g

Healthy Spinach Balls

Servings: 4
Cooking Time: 10 Minutes

Ingredients:
- 1 egg
- 29g breadcrumbs
- ½ medium onion, chopped
- 225g spinach, blanched & chopped
- 1 carrot, peel & grated
- 1 tbsp cornflour
- 1 tbsp nutritional yeast
- 1 tsp garlic, minced
- ½ tsp garlic powder
- Pepper
- Salt

Directions:
1. Add spinach and remaining ingredients into the mixing bowl and mix until well combined.
2. Insert a crisper plate in the Ninja Foodi air fryer baskets.
3. Make small balls from the spinach mixture and place them in both baskets.
4. Select zone 1, then select "air fry" mode and set the temperature to 390 degrees F for 10 minutes. Press "match" to match zone 2 settings to zone 1. Press "start/stop" to begin.

Nutrition Info:

- (Per serving) Calories 74 | Fat 1.7g |Sodium 122mg | Carbs 11.1g | Fiber 1.9g | Sugar 2g | Protein 4.2g

Miso-glazed Shishito Peppers Charred Lemon Shishito Peppers

Servings:4
Cooking Time: 10 Minutes
Ingredients:
- FOR THE MISO-GLAZED PEPPERS
- 2 tablespoons vegetable oil
- 2 tablespoons water
- 1 tablespoon white miso
- 1 teaspoon grated fresh ginger
- ½ pound shishito peppers
- FOR THE CHARRED LEMON PEPPERS
- ½ pound shishito peppers
- 1 lemon, cut into ⅛-inch-thick rounds
- 2 garlic cloves, minced
- 2 tablespoons vegetable oil
- ½ teaspoon kosher salt

Directions:
1. To prep the miso-glazed peppers: In a large bowl, mix the vegetable oil, water, miso, and ginger until well combined. Add the shishitos and toss to coat.
2. To prep the charred lemon peppers: In a large bowl, combine the shishitos, lemon slices, garlic, vegetable oil, and salt. Toss to coat.
3. To cook the peppers: Install a crisper plate in each of the two baskets. Place the miso-glazed peppers in the Zone 1 basket and insert the basket in the unit. Place the peppers with lemons in the Zone 2 basket and insert the basket in the unit.
4. Select Zone 1, select AIR FRY, set the temperature to 390°F, and set the time to 10 minutes. Select MATCH COOK to match Zone 2 settings to Zone 1.
5. Press START/PAUSE to begin cooking.
6. When both timers read 4 minutes, press START/PAUSE. Remove both baskets and shake well. Reinsert the baskets and press START/PAUSE to resume cooking.
7. When cooking is complete, serve immediately.

Nutrition Info:
- (Per serving) Calories: 165; Total fat: 14g; Saturated fat: 2g; Carbohydrates: 9g; Fiber: 2g; Protein: 2g; Sodium: 334mg

Sweet Bites

Servings:4
Cooking Time:12
Ingredients:
- 10 sheets of Phyllo dough, (filo dough)
- 2 tablespoons of melted butter
- 1 cup walnuts, chopped
- 2 teaspoons of honey
- Pinch of cinnamon
- 1 teaspoon of orange zest

Directions:
1. First, layer together 10 Phyllo dough sheets on a flat surface.
2. Then cut it into 4 *4-inch squares.
3. Now, coat the squares with butter, drizzle some honey, orange zest, walnuts, and cinnamon.
4. Bring all 4 corners together and press the corners to make a little like purse design.
5. Divide it amongst air fryer basket and select zone 1 basket using AIR fry mode and set it for 7 minutes at 375 degrees F.
6. Select the MATCH button for the zone 2 basket.
7. Once done, take out and serve.

Nutrition Info:
- (Per serving) Calories 397| Fat 27.1 g| Sodium 271mg | Carbs31.2 g | Fiber 3.2g| Sugar3.3g | Protein 11g

Blueberries Muffins

Servings:2
Cooking Time:15
Ingredients:
- Salt, pinch
- 2 eggs
- 1/3 cup sugar
- 1/3 cup vegetable oil
- 4 tablespoons of water
- 1 teaspoon of lemon zest
- ¼ teaspoon of vanilla extract
- ½ teaspoon of baking powder
- 1 cup all-purpose flour
- 1 cup blueberries

Directions:
1. Take 4 one-cup sized ramekins that are oven safe and layer them with muffin papers.
2. Take a bowl and whisk the egg, sugar, oil, water, vanilla extract, and lemon zest.
3. Whisk it all very well.
4. Now, in a separate bowl, mix the flour, baking powder, and salt.
5. Now, add dry ingredients slowly to wet ingredients.
6. Now, pour this batter into ramekins and top it with blueberries.
7. Now, divide it between both zones of the Ninja Foodie 2-Basket Air Fryer.
8. Set the time for zone 1 to 15 minutes at 350 degrees F.
9. Select the MATCH button for the zone 2 basket.
10. Check if not done, and let it AIR FRY for one more minute.
11. Once it is done, serve.

Nutrition Info:
- (Per serving) Calories 781| Fat41.6g | Sodium 143mg | Carbs 92.7g | Fiber 3.5g| Sugar41.2 g | Protein 0g

Zucchini Chips

Servings: 4
Cooking Time: 15 Minutes
Ingredients:
- 1 medium-sized zucchini
- ½ cup panko breadcrumbs
- ½ teaspoon garlic powder
- ¼ teaspoon onion powder
- 1 egg
- 3 tablespoons flour

Directions:
1. Slice the zucchini into thin slices, about ¼-inch thick.
2. In a mixing bowl, combine the panko breadcrumbs, garlic powder, and onion powder.
3. The egg should be whisked in a different bowl, while the flour should be placed in a third bowl.
4. Dip the zucchini slices in the flour, then in the egg, and finally in the breadcrumbs.
5. Place a crisper plate in each drawer. Put the zucchini slices into each drawer in a single layer. Insert the drawers into the unit.
6. Select zone 1, then AIR FRY, then set the temperature to 360 degrees F/ 180 degrees C with a 6-minute timer. To match zone 2 settings to zone 1, choose MATCH. To begin, select START/STOP.
7. Remove the zucchini from the drawers after the timer has finished.

Nutrition Info:
- (Per serving) Calories 82 | Fat 1.5g | Sodium 89mg | Carbs 14.1g | Fiber 1.7g | Sugar 1.2g | Protein 3.9g

Tofu Veggie Meatballs

Servings: 4
Cooking Time: 10minutes
Ingredients:
- 122g firm tofu, drained
- 50g breadcrumbs
- 37g bamboo shoots, thinly sliced
- 22g carrots, shredded & steamed
- 1 tsp garlic powder
- 1 ½ tbsp soy sauce
- 2 tbsp cornstarch
- 3 dried shitake mushrooms, soaked & chopped
- Pepper
- Salt

Directions:
1. Add tofu and remaining ingredients into the food processor and process until well combined.
2. Insert a crisper plate in the Ninja Foodi air fryer baskets.
3. Make small balls from the tofu mixture and place them in both baskets.
4. Select zone 1, then select "air fry" mode and set the temperature to 380 degrees F for 10 minutes. Press "match" to match zone 2 settings to zone 1. Press "start/stop" to begin. Turn halfway through.

Nutrition Info:
- (Per serving) Calories 125 | Fat 1.8g |Sodium 614mg | Carbs 23.4g | Fiber 2.5g | Sugar 3.8g | Protein 5.3g

Stuffed Bell Peppers

Servings:3
Cooking Time:16
Ingredients:
- 6 large bell peppers
- 1-1/2 cup cooked rice
- 2 cups cheddar cheese

Directions:
1. Cut the bell peppers in half lengthwise and remove all the seeds.
2. Fill the cavity of each bell pepper with cooked rice.
3. Divide the bell peppers amongst the two zones of the air fryer basket.
4. Set the time for zone 1 for 200 degrees for 10 minutes.
5. Select MATCH button of zone 2 basket.
6. Afterward, take out the baskets and sprinkle cheese on top.
7. Set the time for zone 1 for 200 degrees for 6 minutes.
8. Select MATCH button of zone 2 basket.
9. Once it's done, serve.

Nutrition Info:
- (Per serving) Calories 605| Fat 26g | Sodium477 mg | Carbs68.3 g | Fiber4 g| Sugar 12.5g | Protein25.6 g

Fried Ravioli

Servings: 6
Cooking Time: 7 Minutes
Ingredients:
- 12 frozen raviolis
- 118ml buttermilk
- ½ cup Italian breadcrumbs

Directions:
1. Dip the ravioli in the buttermilk then coat with the breadcrumbs.
2. Divide the ravioli into the Ninja Foodi 2 Baskets Air Fryer baskets.
3. Return the air fryer basket 1 to Zone 1, and basket 2 to Zone 2 of the Ninja Foodi 2-Basket Air Fryer.
4. Choose the "Air Fry" mode for Zone 1 and set the temperature to 400 degrees F and 7 minutes of cooking time.
5. Select the "MATCH COOK" option to copy the settings for Zone 2.
6. Initiate cooking by pressing the START/PAUSE BUTTON.
7. Flip the ravioli once cooked halfway through.
8. Serve warm.

Nutrition Info:

- (Per serving) Calories 134 | Fat 5.9g | Sodium 343mg | Carbs 9.5g | Fiber 0.5g | Sugar 1.1g | Protein 10.4g

Tater Tots

Servings: 4
Cooking Time: 8 Minutes
Ingredients:
- 16 ounces tater tots
- ½ cup shredded cheddar cheese
- 1½ teaspoons bacon bits
- 2 green onions, chopped
- Sour cream (optional)

Directions:
1. Place a crisper plate in each drawer. Put the tater tots into the drawers in a single layer. Insert the drawers into the unit.
2. Select zone 1, then AIR FRY, then set the temperature to 360 degrees F/ 180 degrees C with a 6-minute timer. To match zone 2 settings to zone 1, choose MATCH. To begin, select START/STOP.
3. When the cooking time is over, add the shredded cheddar cheese, bacon bits, and green onions over the tater tots. Select zone 1, AIR FRY, 360 degrees F/ 180 degrees C, for 4 minutes. Select MATCH. Press START/STOP.
4. Drizzle sour cream over the top before serving.
5. Enjoy!

Nutrition Info:
- (Per serving) Calories 335 | Fat 19.1g | Sodium 761mg | Carbs 34.1g | Fiber 3g | Sugar 0.6g | Protein 8.9g

Mac And Cheese Balls

Servings: 4
Cooking Time: 20 Minutes
Ingredients:
- 1 cup panko breadcrumbs
- 4 cups prepared macaroni and cheese, refrigerated
- 3 tablespoons flour
- 1 teaspoon salt, divided
- 1 teaspoon ground black pepper, divided
- 1 teaspoon smoked paprika, divided
- ½ teaspoon garlic powder, divided
- 2 eggs
- 1 tablespoon milk
- ¼ cup ranch dressing, garlic aioli, or chipotle mayo, for dipping (optional)

Directions:
1. Preheat a conventional oven to 400 degrees F/ 200 degrees C.
2. Shake the breadcrumbs onto a baking sheet so that they're evenly distributed. Bake in the oven for 3 minutes, then shake and bake for an additional 1 to 2 minutes, or until toasted.
3. Form the chilled macaroni and cheese into golf ball-sized balls and set them aside.
4. Combine the flour, ½ teaspoon salt, ½ teaspoon black pepper, ½ teaspoon smoked paprika, and ¼ teaspoon garlic powder in a large mixing bowl.
5. In a small bowl, whisk together the eggs and milk.
6. Combine the breadcrumbs, remaining salt, pepper, paprika, and garlic powder in a mixing bowl.
7. To coat the macaroni and cheese balls, roll them in the flour mixture, then the egg mixture, and then the breadcrumb mixture.
8. Place a crisper plate in each drawer. Put the cheese balls in a single layer in each drawer. Insert the drawers into the unit.
9. Select zone 1, then AIR FRY, then set the temperature to 360 degrees F/ 180 degrees C with an 8-minute timer. To match zone 2 settings to zone 1, choose MATCH. To begin, select START/STOP.
10. Serve and enjoy!

Nutrition Info:
- (Per serving) Calories 489 | Fat 15.9g | Sodium 1402mg | Carbs 69.7g | Fiber 2.5g | Sugar 4g | Protein 16.9g

Crispy Plantain Chips

Servings: 4
Cooking Time: 20 Minutes.
Ingredients:
- 1 green plantain
- 1 teaspoon canola oil
- ½ teaspoon sea salt

Directions:
1. Peel and cut the plantains into long strips using a mandolin slicer.
2. Grease the crisper plates with ½ teaspoon of canola oil.
3. Toss the plantains with salt and remaining canola oil.
4. Divide these plantains in the two crisper plates.
5. Return the crisper plate to the Ninja Foodi Dual Zone Air Fryer.
6. Choose the Air Fry mode for Zone 1 and set the temperature to 350 degrees F and the time to 20 minutes.
7. Select the "MATCH" button to copy the settings for Zone 2.
8. Initiate cooking by pressing the START/STOP button.
9. Toss the plantains after 10 minutes and resume cooking.
10. Serve warm.

Nutrition Info:
- (Per serving) Calories 122 | Fat 1.8g | Sodium 794mg | Carbs 17g | Fiber 8.9g | Sugar 1.6g | Protein 14.9g

Fried Cheese

Servings: 4
Cooking Time: 12 Minutes
Ingredients:
- 1 Mozzarella cheese block, cut into sticks
- 2 teaspoons olive oil

Directions:
1. Divide the cheese slices into the Ninja Foodi 2 Baskets Air Fryer baskets.
2. Drizzle olive oil over the cheese slices.
3. Return the air fryer basket 1 to Zone 1, and basket 2 to Zone 2 of the Ninja Foodi 2-Basket Air Fryer.
4. Choose the "Air Fry" mode for Zone 1 and set the temperature to 360 degrees F and 12 minutes of cooking time.
5. Flip the cheese slices once cooked halfway through.
6. Serve.

Nutrition Info:
- (Per serving) Calories 186 | Fat 3g |Sodium 223mg | Carbs 31g | Fiber 8.7g | Sugar 5.5g | Protein 9.7g

Potato Chips

Servings: 4
Cooking Time: 16 Minutes
Ingredients:
- 2 large potatoes, peeled and sliced
- 1½ teaspoons salt
- 1½ teaspoons black pepper
- Oil for misting

Directions:
1. Soak potatoes in cold water for 30 minutes then drain.
2. Pat dry the potato slices and toss them with cracked pepper, salt and oil mist.
3. Spread the potatoes in the air fryer basket.
4. Return the air fryer basket 1 to Zone 1, and basket 2 to Zone 2 of the Ninja Foodi 2-Basket Air Fryer.
5. Choose the "Air Fry" mode for Zone 1 at 300 degrees F and 16 minutes of cooking time.
6. Select the "MATCH COOK" option to copy the settings for Zone 2.
7. Initiate cooking by pressing the START/PAUSE BUTTON.
8. Toss the fries once cooked halfway through.
9. Serve warm.

Nutrition Info:
- (Per serving) Calories 122 | Fat 1.8g |Sodium 794mg | Carbs 17g | Fiber 8.9g | Sugar 1.6g | Protein 14.9g

"fried" Ravioli With Zesty Marinara

Servings: 6
Cooking Time: 20 Minutes
Ingredients:
- FOR THE RAVIOLI
- ¼ cup all-purpose flour
- 1 large egg
- 1 tablespoon water
- ⅔ cup Italian-style bread crumbs
- 1 pound frozen cheese ravioli, thawed
- Nonstick cooking spray
- FOR THE MARINARA
- 1 (28-ounce) can chunky crushed tomatoes with basil and oregano
- 1 tablespoon unsalted butter
- 2 garlic cloves, minced
- ¼ teaspoon kosher salt
- ¼ teaspoon red pepper flakes

Directions:
1. To prep the ravioli: Set up a breading station with three small shallow bowls. Put the flour in the first bowl. In the second bowl, beat the egg and water. Place the bread crumbs in the third bowl.
2. Bread the ravioli in this order: First dip them into the flour, coating both sides. Then dip into the beaten egg. Finally, coat them in the bread crumbs, gently pressing the crumbs into the ravioli to help them stick.
3. Mist both sides of the ravioli generously with cooking spray.
4. To prep the marinara: In the Zone 2 basket, combine the crushed tomatoes, butter, garlic, salt, and red pepper flakes.
5. To cook the ravioli and sauce: Install a crisper plate in the Zone 1 basket and add the ravioli to the basket. Insert the basket in the unit. Insert the Zone 2 basket in the unit.
6. Select Zone 1, select AIR FRY, set the temperature to 390°F, and set the time to 20 minutes.
7. Select Zone 2, select BAKE, set the temperature to 350°F, and set the time to 15 minutes. Select SMART FINISH.
8. Press START/PAUSE to begin cooking.
9. When the Zone 1 timer reads 7 minutes, press START/PAUSE. Remove the basket and shake to redistribute the ravioli. Reinsert the basket and press START/PAUSE to resume cooking.
10. When cooking is complete, the breading will be crisp and golden brown. Transfer the ravioli to a plate and the marinara to a bowl. Serve hot.

Nutrition Info:
- (Per serving) Calories: 282; Total fat: 8g; Saturated fat: 3g; Carbohydrates: 39g; Fiber: 4.5g; Protein: 13g; Sodium: 369mg

Mozzarella Balls

Servings: 6
Cooking Time: 13 Minutes
Ingredients:
- 2 cups mozzarella, shredded
- 3 tablespoons cornstarch
- 3 tablespoons water
- 2 eggs, beaten
- 1 cup Italian seasoned breadcrumbs
- 1 tablespoon Italian seasoning
- 1½ teaspoons garlic powder
- 1 teaspoon salt
- 1½ teaspoons Parmesan

Directions:
1. Mix mozzarella with parmesan, water and cornstarch in a bowl.
2. Make 1-inch balls out of this mixture.
3. Mix breadcrumbs with seasoning, salt, and garlic powder in a bowl.
4. Dip the balls into the beaten eggs and coat with the breadcrumbs.
5. Place the coated balls in the air fryer baskets.
6. Return the air fryer basket 1 to Zone 1, and basket 2 to Zone 2 of the Ninja Foodi 2-Basket Air Fryer.
7. Choose the "Air Fry" mode for Zone 1 and set the temperature to 360 degrees F and 13 minutes of cooking time.
8. Select the "MATCH COOK" option to copy the settings for Zone 2.
9. Initiate cooking by pressing the START/PAUSE BUTTON.
10. Toss the balls once cooked halfway through.
11. Serve.

Nutrition Info:
- (Per serving) Calories 307 | Fat 8.6g |Sodium 510mg | Carbs 22.2g | Fiber 1.4g | Sugar 13g | Protein 33.6g

Chili-lime Crispy Chickpeas
Pizza-seasoned Crispy Chickpeas

Servings:6
Cooking Time: 20 Minutes
Ingredients:
- FOR THE CHILI-LIME CHICKPEAS
- 1½ cups canned chickpeas, rinsed and drained
- ¼ cup fresh lime juice
- 1 tablespoon olive oil
- 1½ teaspoons chili powder
- ½ teaspoon kosher salt
- FOR THE PIZZA-SEASONED CHICKPEAS
- 1½ cups canned chickpeas, rinsed and drained
- 1 tablespoon olive oil
- 1 tablespoon grated Parmesan cheese
- ½ teaspoon dried basil
- ½ teaspoon dried oregano
- ½ teaspoon kosher salt
- ¼ teaspoon onion powder
- ¼ teaspoon garlic powder
- ¼ teaspoon fennel seeds
- ¼ teaspoon dried thyme
- ¼ teaspoon red pepper flakes (optional)

Directions:
1. To prep the chili-lime chickpeas: In a small bowl, mix the chickpeas, lime juice, olive oil, chili powder, and salt until the chickpeas are well coated.
2. To prep the pizza-seasoned chickpeas: In a small bowl, mix the chickpeas, olive oil, Parmesan, basil, oregano, salt, onion powder, garlic powder, fennel, thyme, and red pepper flakes (if using) until the chickpeas are well coated.
3. To cook the chickpeas: Install a crisper plate in each of the two baskets. Place the chili-lime chickpeas in the Zone 1 basket and insert the basket in the unit. Place the pizza-seasoned chickpeas in the Zone 2 basket and insert the basket in the unit.
4. Select Zone 1, select AIR FRY, set the temperature to 375°F, and set the time to 20 minutes. Select MATCH COOK to match Zone 2 settings to Zone 1.
5. Press START/PAUSE to begin cooking.
6. When both timers read 10 minutes, press START/PAUSE. Remove both baskets and give each basket a shake to redistribute the chickpeas. Reinsert both baskets and press START/PAUSE to resume cooking.
7. When both timers read 5 minutes, press START/PAUSE. Remove both baskets and give each basket a good shake again. Reinsert both baskets and press START/PAUSE to resume cooking.
8. When cooking is complete, the chickpeas will be crisp and golden brown. Serve warm or at room temperature.

Nutrition Info:
- (Per serving) Calories: 145; Total fat: 6.5g; Saturated fat: 0.5g; Carbohydrates: 17g; Fiber: 4.5g; Protein: 5g; Sodium: 348mg

Tasty Sweet Potato Wedges

Servings: 4
Cooking Time: 20 Minutes
Ingredients:
- 2 sweet potatoes, peel & cut into wedges
- 1 tbsp BBQ spice rub
- ½ tsp sweet paprika
- 1 tbsp olive oil
- Pepper
- Salt

Directions:
1. In a bowl, toss sweet potato wedges with sweet paprika, oil, BBQ spice rub, pepper, and salt.

2. Insert a crisper plate in the Ninja Foodi air fryer baskets.
3. Add sweet potato wedges in both baskets.
4. Select zone 1 then select "air fry" mode and set the temperature to 390 degrees F for 20 minutes. Press "match" to match zone 2 settings to zone 1. Press "start/stop" to begin. Turn halfway through.

Nutrition Info:
- (Per serving) Calories 87 | Fat 3.6g |Sodium 75mg | Carbs 13.2g | Fiber 2.1g | Sugar 2.8g | Protein 1.1g

Kale Potato Nuggets

Servings: 4
Cooking Time: 15minutes

Ingredients:
- 279g potatoes, chopped, boiled & mashed
- 268g kale, chopped
- 1 garlic clove, minced
- 30ml milk
- Pepper
- Salt

Directions:
1. In a bowl, mix potatoes, kale, milk, garlic, pepper, and salt until well combined.
2. Insert a crisper plate in the Ninja Foodi air fryer baskets.
3. Make small balls from the potato mixture and place them both baskets.
4. Select zone 1 then select "air fry" mode and set the temperature to 390 degrees F for 15 minutes. Press "match" to match zone 2 settings to zone 1. Press "start/stop" to begin. Turn halfway through.

Nutrition Info:
- (Per serving) Calories 90 | Fat 0.2g |Sodium 76mg | Carbs 19.4g | Fiber 2.8g | Sugar 1.2g | Protein 3.6g

Crab Rangoon Dip With Crispy Wonton Strips

Servings:6
Cooking Time: 15 Minutes

Ingredients:
- FOR THE DIP
- 1 (6-ounce) can pink crab, drained
- 8 ounces (16 tablespoons) cream cheese, at room temperature
- ½ cup sour cream
- 1 tablespoon chopped scallions
- ½ teaspoon garlic powder
- 1 teaspoon Worcestershire sauce
- ¼ teaspoon kosher salt
- 1 cup shredded part-skim mozzarella cheese
- FOR THE WONTON STRIPS
- 12 wonton wrappers
- 1 tablespoon olive oil
- ¼ teaspoon kosher salt

Directions:
1. To prep the dip: In a medium bowl, mix the crab, cream cheese, sour cream, scallions, garlic powder, Worcestershire sauce, and salt until smooth.
2. To prep the wonton strips: Brush both sides of the wonton wrappers with the oil and sprinkle with salt. Cut the wonton wrappers into ¾-inch-wide strips.
3. To cook the dip and strips: Pour the dip into the Zone 1 basket, top with the mozzarella cheese, and insert the basket in the unit. Install a crisper plate in the Zone 2 basket, add the wonton strips, and insert the basket in the unit.
4. Select Zone 1, select BAKE, set the temperature to 330°F, and set the time to 15 minutes.
5. Select Zone 2, select AIR FRY, set the temperature to 350°F, and set the time to 6 minutes. Select SMART FINISH.
6. Press START/PAUSE to begin cooking.
7. When the Zone 2 timer reads 4 minutes, press START/PAUSE. Remove the basket and shake well to redistribute the wonton strips. Reinsert the basket and press START/PAUSE to resume cooking.
8. When the Zone 2 timer reads 2 minutes, press START/PAUSE. Remove the basket and shake well to redistribute the wonton strips. Reinsert the basket and press START/PAUSE to resume cooking.
9. When cooking is complete, the dip will be bubbling and golden brown on top and the wonton strips will be crunchy. Serve warm.

Nutrition Info:
- (Per serving) Calories: 315; Total fat: 23g; Saturated fat: 12g; Carbohydrates: 14g; Fiber: 0.5g; Protein: 14g; Sodium: 580mg

Cinnamon Sugar Chickpeas

Servings: 4
Cooking Time: 15 Minutes

Ingredients:
- 2 cups chickpeas, drained
- Spray oil
- 1 tablespoon coconut sugar
- ½ teaspoon cinnamon
- Serving
- 57g cheddar cheese, cubed
- ¼ cup raw almonds
- 85g jerky, sliced

Directions:
1. Toss chickpeas with coconut sugar, cinnamon and oil in a bowl.
2. Divide the chickpeas into the Ninja Foodi 2 Baskets Air Fryer baskets.
3. Drizzle cheddar cheese, almonds and jerky on top.
4. Return the air fryer basket 1 to Zone 1, and basket 2 to Zone 2 of the Ninja Foodi 2-Basket Air Fryer.
5. Choose the "Air Fry" mode for Zone 1 at 380 degrees F and 15 minutes of cooking time.

6. Select the "MATCH COOK" option to copy the settings for Zone 2.
7. Initiate cooking by pressing the START/PAUSE BUTTON.
8. Toss the chickpeas once cooked halfway through.
9. Serve warm.

Nutrition Info:
- (Per serving) Calories 103 | Fat 8.4g |Sodium 117mg | Carbs 3.5g | Fiber 0.9g | Sugar 1.5g | Protein 5.1g

Dried Apple Chips Dried Banana Chips

Servings:6
Cooking Time: 6 To 10 Hours
Ingredients:
- FOR THE APPLE CHIPS
- ½ teaspoon ground cinnamon
- ¼ teaspoon ground nutmeg
- ⅛ teaspoon ground allspice
- ⅛ teaspoon ground ginger
- 2 Gala apples, cored and cut into ⅛-inch-thick rings
- FOR THE BANANA CHIPS
- 2 firm-ripe bananas, cut into ¼-inch slices

Directions:
1. To prep the apple chips: In a small bowl, mix the cinnamon, nutmeg, allspice, and ginger until combined. Sprinkle the spice mixture over the apple slices.
2. To dehydrate the fruit: Arrange half of the apple slices in a single layer in the Zone 1 basket. It is okay if the edges overlap a bit as they will shrink as they cook. Place a crisper plate on top of the apples. Arrange the remaining apple slices on top of the crisper plate and insert the basket in the unit.
3. Repeat this process with the bananas in the Zone 2 basket and insert the basket in the unit.
4. Select Zone 1, select DEHYDRATE, set the temperature to 135°F, and set the time to 8 hours.
5. Select Zone 2, select DEHYDRATE, set the temperature to 135°F, and set the time to 10 hours. Select SMART FINISH.
6. Press START/PAUSE to begin cooking.
7. When both timers read 2 hours, press START/PAUSE. Remove both baskets and check the fruit for doneness; note that juicier fruit will take longer to dry than fruit that starts out drier. Reinsert the basket and press START/PAUSE to continue cooking if necessary.

Nutrition Info:
- (Per serving) Calories: 67; Total fat: 0g; Saturated fat: 0g; Carbohydrates: 16g; Fiber: 3g; Protein: 0g; Sodium: 1mg

Parmesan Crush Chicken

Servings:4
Cooking Time:18
Ingredients:
- 4 chicken breasts
- 1 cup parmesan cheese
- 1 cup bread crumb
- 2 eggs, whisked
- Salt, to taste
- Oil spray, for greasing

Directions:
1. Whisk egg in a large bowl and set aside.
2. Season the chicken breast with salt and then put it in egg wash.
3. Next, dredge it in breadcrumb then parmesan cheese.
4. Line both the basket of the air fryer with parchment paper.
5. Divided the breast pieces between the backsets, and oil spray the breast pieces.
6. Set zone 1 basket to air fry mode at 350 degrees F for 18 minutes.
7. Select the MATCH button for the zone 2 basket.
8. Once it's done, serve.

Nutrition Info:
- (Per serving) Calories574 | Fat25g | Sodium848 mg | Carbs 21.4g | Fiber 1.2g| Sugar 1.8g | Protein 64.4g

Roasted Tomato Bruschetta With Toasty Garlic Bread

Servings:4
Cooking Time: 12 Minutes
Ingredients:
- FOR THE ROASTED TOMATOES
- 10 ounces cherry tomatoes, cut in half
- 1 tablespoon balsamic vinegar
- 1 tablespoon olive oil
- ¼ teaspoon kosher salt
- ¼ teaspoon freshly ground black pepper
- FOR THE GARLIC BREAD
- 4 slices crusty Italian bread
- 1 tablespoon olive oil
- 3 garlic cloves, minced
- ¼ teaspoon Italian seasoning
- FOR THE BRUSCHETTA
- ¼ cup loosely packed fresh basil, thinly sliced
- ½ cup part-skim ricotta cheese

Directions:
1. To prep the tomatoes: In a small bowl, combine the tomatoes, vinegar, oil, salt, and black pepper.
2. To prep the garlic bread: Brush one side of each bread slice with the oil. Sprinkle with the garlic and Italian seasoning.
3. To cook the tomatoes and garlic bread: Install a broil rack in the Zone 1 basket (without the crisper plate installed). Place the tomatoes on the rack in the basket and insert the basket in the unit.
4. Place 2 slices of bread in the Zone 2 basket and insert the basket in the unit.

5. Select Zone 1, select AIR BROIL, set the temperature to 450°F, and set the time to 12 minutes.
6. Select Zone 2, select AIR FRY, set the temperature to 360°F, and set the time to 10 minutes. Select SMART FINISH.
7. Press START/PAUSE to begin cooking.
8. When the Zone 2 timer reads 5 minutes, press START/PAUSE. Remove the basket and transfer the garlic bread to a cutting board. Place the remaining 2 slices of garlic bread in the basket. Reinsert the basket in the unit and press START/PAUSE to resume cooking.
9. To assemble the bruschetta: When cooking is complete, add the basil to the tomatoes and stir to combine. Spread 2 tablespoons of ricotta onto each slice of garlic bread and top with the tomatoes. Serve warm or at room temperature.

Nutrition Info:
- (Per serving) Calories: 212; Total fat: 11g; Saturated fat: 2.5g; Carbohydrates: 22g; Fiber: 1.5g; Protein: 6g; Sodium: 286mg

Fish And Seafood Recipes

Breaded Scallops

Servings: 4
Cooking Time: 12 Minutes.

Ingredients:
- ½ cup crushed buttery crackers
- ½ teaspoon garlic powder
- ½ teaspoon seafood seasoning
- 2 tablespoons butter, melted
- 1 pound sea scallops patted dry
- cooking spray

Directions:
1. Mix cracker crumbs, garlic powder, and seafood seasoning in a shallow bowl. Spread melted butter in another shallow bowl.
2. Dip each scallop in the melted butter and then roll in the breading to coat well.
3. Grease each Air fryer basket with cooking spray and place half of the scallops in each.
4. Return the crisper plate to the Ninja Foodi Dual Zone Air Fryer.
5. Select the Air Fry mode for Zone 1 and set the temperature to 390 degrees F and the time to 12 minutes.
6. Press the "MATCH" button to copy the settings for Zone 2.
7. Initiate cooking by pressing the START/STOP button.
8. Flip the scallops with a spatula after 4 minutes and resume cooking.
9. Serve warm.

Nutrition Info:
- (Per serving) Calories 275 | Fat 1.4g |Sodium 582mg | Carbs 31.5g | Fiber 1.1g | Sugar 0.1g | Protein 29.8g

Seafood Shrimp Omelet

Servings: 2
Cooking Time: 15

Ingredients:
- 6 large shrimp, shells removed and chopped
- 6 eggs, beaten
- ½ tablespoon of butter, melted
- 2 tablespoons green onions, sliced
- 1/3 cup of mushrooms, chopped
- 1 pinch paprika
- Salt and black pepper, to taste
- Oil spray, for greasing

Directions:
1. In a large bowl whisk the eggs and add chopped shrimp, butter, green onions, mushrooms, paprika, salt, and black pepper.
2. Take two cake pans that fit inside the air fryer and grease them with oil spray.
3. Pour the egg mixture between the cake pans and place it in two baskets of the air fryer.
4. Turn on the BAKE function of zone 1, and let it cook for 15 minutes at 320 degrees F.
5. Select the MATCH button to match the cooking time for the zone 2 basket.
6. Once the cooking cycle completes, take out, and serve hot.

Nutrition Info:
- (Per serving) Calories 300 | Fat 17.5g| Sodium 368mg | Carbs 2.9g | Fiber 0.3g | Sugar 1.4 g | Protein 32.2 g

Crispy Catfish

Servings: 4
Cooking Time: 17 Minutes.
Ingredients:
- 4 catfish fillets
- ¼ cup Louisiana Fish fry
- 1 tablespoon olive oil
- 1 tablespoon parsley, chopped
- 1 lemon, sliced
- Fresh herbs, to garnish

Directions:
1. Mix fish fry with olive oil, and parsley then liberally rub over the catfish.
2. Place two fillets in each of the crisper plate.
3. Return the crisper plates to the Ninja Foodi Dual Zone Air Fryer.
4. Choose the Air Fry mode for Zone 1 and set the temperature to 390 degrees F and the time to 17 minutes.
5. Select the "MATCH" button to copy the settings for Zone 2.
6. Initiate cooking by pressing the START/STOP button.
7. Garnish with lemon slices and herbs.
8. Serve warm.

Nutrition Info:
- (Per serving) Calories 275 | Fat 1.4g |Sodium 582mg | Carbs 31.5g | Fiber 1.1g | Sugar 0.1g | Protein 29.8g

Codfish With Herb Vinaigrette

Servings: 2
Cooking Time: 16
Ingredients:
- Vinaigrette Ingredients:
- 1/2 cup parsley leaves
- 1 cup basil leaves
- ½ cup mint leaves
- 2 tablespoons thyme leaves
- 1/4 teaspoon red pepper flakes
- 2 cloves of garlic
- 4 tablespoons of red wine vinegar
- ¼ cup of olive oil
- Salt, to taste
- Other Ingredients:
- 1.5 pounds fish fillets, cod fish
- 2 tablespoons olive oil
- Salt and black pepper, to taste
- 1 teaspoon of paprika
- 1teasbpoon of Italian seasoning

Directions:
1. Blend the entire vinaigrette ingredient in a high-speed blender and pulse into a smooth paste.
2. Set aside for drizzling overcooked fish.
3. Rub the fillets with salt, black pepper, paprika, Italian seasoning, and olive oil.
4. Divide it between two baskets of the air fryer.
5. Set the zone 1 to 16 minutes at 390 degrees F, at AIR FRY mode.
6. Press the MATCH button for the second basket.
7. Once done, serve the fillets with the drizzle of blended vinaigrette

Nutrition Info:
- (Per serving) Calories 1219| Fat 81.8g| Sodium 1906mg | Carbs64.4 g | Fiber5.5 g | Sugar 0.4g | Protein 52.1g

Bang Bang Shrimp With Roasted Bok Choy

Servings: 4
Cooking Time: 13 Minutes
Ingredients:
- FOR THE BANG BANG SHRIMP
- ½ cup all-purpose flour
- 2 large eggs
- 1 cup panko bread crumbs
- 1 pound peeled shrimp (tails removed), thawed if frozen
- Nonstick cooking spray
- ½ cup mayonnaise
- ¼ cup Thai sweet chili sauce
- ¼ teaspoon sriracha
- FOR THE BOK CHOY
- 1 tablespoon reduced-sodium soy sauce
- 1 teaspoon minced garlic
- 1 teaspoon sesame oil
- 1 teaspoon minced fresh ginger
- 1½ pounds baby bok choy, halved lengthwise
- 1 tablespoon toasted sesame seeds

Directions:
1. To prep the shrimp: Set up a breading station with three small shallow bowls. Place the flour in the first bowl. In the second bowl, whisk the eggs. Place the panko in the third bowl.
2. Bread the shrimp in this order: First, dip them into the flour, coating both sides. Then, dip into the beaten egg. Finally, coat them in the panko, gently pressing the bread crumbs to adhere to the shrimp. Spritz both sides of the shrimp with cooking spray.
3. To prep the bok choy: In a small bowl, whisk together the soy sauce, garlic, sesame oil, and ginger.
4. To cook the shrimp and bok choy: Install a crisper plate in the Zone 1 basket. Place the shrimp in the basket in a single layer and insert the basket in the unit. Place the boy choy cut-side up in the Zone 2 basket. Pour the sauce over the bok choy and insert the basket in the unit.
5. Select Zone 1, select AIR FRY, set the temperature to 390°F, and set the timer to 13 minutes.

6. Select Zone 2, select BAKE, set the temperature to 370°F, and set the timer to 8 minutes. Select SMART FINISH.
7. Press START/PAUSE to begin cooking.
8. When cooking is complete, the shrimp should be cooked through and golden brown and the bok choy soft and slightly caramelized.
9. In a large bowl, whisk together the mayonnaise, sweet chili sauce, and sriracha. Add the shrimp and toss to coat.
10. Sprinkle the bok choy with the sesame seeds and serve hot alongside the shrimp.

Nutrition Info:
- (Per serving) Calories: 534; Total fat: 33g; Saturated fat: 4g; Carbohydrates: 29g; Fiber: 3g; Protein: 31g; Sodium: 789mg

Fried Tilapia

Servings: 4
Cooking Time: 20 Minutes
Ingredients:
- 4 fresh tilapia fillets, approximately 6 ounces each
- 2 teaspoons olive oil
- 2 teaspoons chopped fresh chives
- 2 teaspoons chopped fresh parsley
- 1 teaspoon minced garlic
- Freshly ground pepper, to taste
- Salt to taste

Directions:
1. Pat the tilapia fillets dry with a paper towel.
2. Stir together the olive oil, chives, parsley, garlic, salt, and pepper in a small bowl.
3. Brush the mixture over the top of the tilapia fillets.
4. Place a crisper plate in each drawer. Add the fillets in a single layer to each drawer. Insert the drawers into the unit.
5. Select zone 1, then AIR FRY, then set the temperature to 360 degrees F/ 180 degrees C with a 20-minute timer. To match zone 2 settings to zone 1, choose MATCH. To begin, select START/STOP.
6. Remove the tilapia fillets from the drawers after the timer has finished.

Nutrition Info:
- (Per serving) Calories 140 | Fat 5.7g | Sodium 125mg | Carbs 1.5g | Fiber 0.4g | Sugar 0g | Protein 21.7g

Spicy Salmon Fillets

Servings: 6
Cooking Time: 8 Minutes
Ingredients:
- 900g salmon fillets
- ¾ tsp ground cumin
- 1 tbsp brown sugar
- 2 tbsp steak seasoning
- ¼ tsp cayenne pepper
- ½ tsp ground coriander

Directions:
1. Mix ground cumin, coriander, steak seasoning, brown sugar, and cayenne in a small bowl.
2. Rub salmon fillets with spice mixture.
3. Insert a crisper plate in the Ninja Foodi air fryer baskets.
4. Place the salmon fillets in both baskets.
5. Select zone 1, then select "bake" mode and set the temperature to 360 degrees F for 10 minutes. Press "match" to match zone 2 settings to zone 1. Press "start/stop" to begin.

Nutrition Info:
- (Per serving) Calories 207 | Fat 9.4g |Sodium 68mg | Carbs 1.6g | Fiber 0.1g | Sugar 1.5g | Protein 29.4g

Salmon Patties

Servings: 8
Cooking Time: 18 Minutes.
Ingredients:
- 1 lb. fresh Atlantic salmon side
- ¼ cup avocado, mashed
- ¼ cup cilantro, diced
- 1 ½ teaspoons yellow curry powder
- ½ teaspoons sea salt
- ¼ cup, 4 teaspoons tapioca starch
- 2 brown eggs
- ½ cup coconut flakes
- Coconut oil, melted, for brushing
- For the greens:
- 2 teaspoons organic coconut oil, melted
- 6 cups arugula & spinach mix, tightly packed
- Pinch of sea salt

Directions:
1. Remove the fish skin and dice the flesh.
2. Place in a large bowl. Add cilantro, avocado, salt, and curry powder mix gently.
3. Add tapioca starch and mix well again.
4. Make 8 salmon patties out of this mixture, about a half-inch thick.
5. Place them on a baking sheet lined with wax paper and freeze them for 20 minutes.
6. Place ¼ cup tapioca starch and coconut flakes on a flat plate.
7. Dip the patties in the whisked egg, then coat the frozen patties in the starch and flakes.
8. Place half of the patties in each of the crisper plate and spray them with cooking oil
9. Return the crisper plate to the Ninja Foodi Dual Zone Air Fryer.
10. Choose the Air Fry mode for Zone 1 and set the temperature to 390 degrees F and the time to 17 minutes.
11. Select the "MATCH" button to copy the settings for Zone 2.
12. Initiate cooking by pressing the START/STOP button.

13. Flip the patties once cooked halfway through, then resume cooking.
14. Sauté arugula with spinach in coconut oil in a pan for 30 seconds.
15. Serve the patties with sautéed greens mixture

Nutrition Info:
- (Per serving) Calories 260 | Fat 16g | Sodium 585mg | Carbs 3.1g | Fiber 1.3g | Sugar 0.2g | Protein 25.5g

Foil Packet Salmon

Servings: 4
Cooking Time: 14 Minutes
Ingredients:
- 455g salmon fillets
- 4 cups green beans defrosted
- 4 tablespoons soy sauce
- 2 tablespoons honey
- 2 teaspoons sesame seeds
- 1 teaspoon garlic powder
- ½ teaspoon ginger powder
- ½ teaspoon salt
- ¼ teaspoon white pepper
- ¼ teaspoon red pepper flakes
- Salt, to taste
- Canola oil spray

Directions:
1. Make 4 foil packets and adjust the salmon fillets in each.
2. Divide the green beans in the foil packets and drizzle half of the spices on top.
3. Place one salmon piece on top of each and drizzle the remaining ingredients on top.
4. Pack the salmon with the foil and place two packets in each air fryer basket.
5. Return the air fryer basket 1 to Zone 1, and basket 2 to Zone 2 of the Ninja Foodi 2-Basket Air Fryer.
6. Choose the "Air Fry" mode for Zone 1 and set the temperature to 425 degrees F and 14 minutes of cooking time.
7. Select the "MATCH COOK" option to copy the settings for Zone 2.
8. Initiate cooking by pressing the START/PAUSE BUTTON.
9. Serve warm.

Nutrition Info:
- (Per serving) Calories 305 | Fat 15g | Sodium 482mg | Carbs 17g | Fiber 3g | Sugar 2g | Protein 35g

Lemon Pepper Fish Fillets

Servings: 4
Cooking Time: 10 Minutes
Ingredients:
- 4 tilapia fillets
- 30ml olive oil
- 2 tbsp lemon zest
- ⅛ tsp paprika
- 1 tsp garlic, minced
- 1 ½ tsp ground peppercorns
- Pepper
- Salt

Directions:
1. In a small bowl, mix oil, peppercorns, paprika, garlic, lemon zest, pepper, and salt.
2. Brush the fish fillets with oil mixture.
3. Insert a crisper plate in the Ninja Foodi air fryer baskets.
4. Place fish fillets in both baskets.
5. Select zone 1 then select "air fry" mode and set the temperature to 390 degrees F for 10 minutes. Press "match" to match zone 2 settings to zone 1. Press "start/stop" to begin.

Nutrition Info:
- (Per serving) Calories 203 | Fat 9g | Sodium 99mg | Carbs 0.9g | Fiber 0.2g | Sugar 0.2g | Protein 32.1g

Buttered Mahi-mahi

Servings: 4
Cooking Time: 22 Minutes.
Ingredients:
- 4 (6-oz) mahi-mahi fillets
- Salt and black pepper ground to taste
- Cooking spray
- ⅔ cup butter

Directions:
1. Preheat your Ninja Foodi Dual Zone Air Fryer to 350 degrees F.
2. Rub the mahi-mahi fillets with salt and black pepper.
3. Place two mahi-mahi fillets in each of the crisper plate.
4. Return the crisper plates to the Ninja Foodi Dual Zone Air Fryer.
5. Choose the Air Fry mode for Zone 1 and set the temperature to 390 degrees F and the time to 17 minutes.
6. Select the "MATCH" button to copy the settings for Zone 2.
7. Initiate cooking by pressing the START/STOP button.
8. Add butter to a saucepan and cook for 5 minutes until slightly brown.
9. Remove the butter from the heat.
10. Drizzle butter over the fish and serve warm.

Nutrition Info:
- (Per serving) Calories 399 | Fat 16g | Sodium 537mg | Carbs 28g | Fiber 3g | Sugar 10g | Protein 35g

Crusted Shrimp

Servings: 4
Cooking Time: 13 Minutes.
Ingredients:
- 1 lb. shrimp
- ½ cup flour, all-purpose
- 1 teaspoon salt

- ½ teaspoon baking powder
- ⅔ cup water
- 2 cups coconut shred
- ½ cup bread crumbs

Directions:
1. In a small bowl, whisk together flour, salt, water, and baking powder. Set aside for 5 minutes.
2. In another shallow bowl, toss bread crumbs with coconut shreds together.
3. Dredge shrimp in liquid, then coat in coconut mixture, making sure it's totally covered.
4. Repeat until all shrimp are coated.
5. Spread half of the shrimp in each crisper plate and spray them with cooking oil.
6. Return the crisper plates to the Ninja Foodi Dual Zone Air Fryer.
7. Choose the Air Fry mode for Zone 1 and set the temperature to 390 degrees F and the time to 13 minutes.
8. Select the "MATCH" button to copy the settings for Zone 2.
9. Initiate cooking by pressing the START/STOP button.
10. Shake the baskets once cooked halfway, then resume cooking.
11. Serve with your favorite dip.

Nutrition Info:
- (Per serving) Calories 297 | Fat 1g |Sodium 291mg | Carbs 35g | Fiber 1g | Sugar 9g | Protein 29g

Fish And Chips

Servings:2
Cooking Time:22
Ingredients:
- 1 pound of potatoes, cut lengthwise
- 1 cup seasoned flour
- 2 eggs, organic
- 1/3 cup buttermilk
- 2 cup seafood fry mix
- ½ cup bread crumbs
- 2 codfish fillet, 6 ounces each
- Oil spray, for greasing

Directions:
1. take a bowl and whisk eggs in it along buttermilk.
2. In a separate bowl mix seafood fry mix and bread crumbs
3. Take a baking tray and spread flour on it
4. Dip the fillets first in egg wash, then in flour, and at the end coat it with breadcrumbs mixture.
5. Put the fish fillet in air fryer zone 1 basket.
6. Grease the fish fillet with oil spray.
7. Set zone 1 to AIR FRY mode at 400 degrees F for 14 minutes.
8. Put potato chip in zone two baskets and lightly grease it with oil spray.
9. Set the zone 2 basket to AIRFRY mode at 400 degrees F for 22 minutes.
10. Hit the smart finish button.
11. Once done, serve and enjoy.

Nutrition Info:
- (Per serving) Calories 992| Fat 22.3g| Sodium1406 mg | Carbs 153.6g | Fiber 10g | Sugar10 g | Protein 40g

Cajun Scallops

Servings: 6
Cooking Time: 6 Minutes
Ingredients:
- 6 sea scallops
- Cooking spray
- Salt to taste
- Cajun seasoning

Directions:
1. Season the scallops with Cajun seasoning and salt.
2. Place them in one air fryer basket and spray them with cooking oil.
3. Return the air fryer basket 1 to Zone 1 of the Ninja Foodi 2-Basket Air Fryer.
4. Choose the "Air Fry" mode for Zone 1 and set the temperature to 400 degrees F and 6 minutes of cooking time.
5. Initiate cooking by pressing the START/PAUSE BUTTON.
6. Flip the scallops once cooked halfway through.
7. Serve warm.

Nutrition Info:
- (Per serving) Calories 266 | Fat 6.3g |Sodium 193mg | Carbs 39.1g | Fiber 7.2g | Sugar 5.2g | Protein 14.8g

Bacon-wrapped Shrimp

Servings: 8
Cooking Time: 10 Minutes
Ingredients:
- 24 jumbo raw shrimp, deveined with tail on, fresh or thawed from frozen
- 8 slices bacon, cut into thirds
- 1 tablespoon olive oil
- 1 teaspoon paprika
- 1–2 cloves minced garlic
- 1 tablespoon finely chopped fresh parsley

Directions:
1. Combine the olive oil, paprika, garlic, and parsley in a small bowl.
2. If necessary, peel the raw shrimp, leaving the tails on.
3. Add the shrimp to the oil mixture. Toss to coat well.
4. Wrap a piece of bacon around the middle of each shrimp and place seam-side down on a small baking dish.
5. Refrigerate for 30 minutes before cooking.
6. Place a crisper plate in each drawer. Put the shrimp in a single layer in each drawer. Insert the drawers into the unit.

7. Select zone 1, then AIR FRY, then set the temperature to 360 degrees F/ 180 degrees C with a 10-minute timer. To match zone 2 settings to zone 1, choose MATCH. To begin, select START/STOP.
8. Remove the shrimp from the drawers when the cooking time is over.
Nutrition Info:
- (Per serving) Calories 479 | Fat 15.7g | Sodium 949mg | Carbs 0.6g | Fiber 0.1g | Sugar 0g | Protein 76.1g

Salmon Nuggets

Servings: 4
Cooking Time: 15 Minutes.
Ingredients:
- ⅓ cup maple syrup
- ¼ teaspoon dried chipotle pepper
- 1 pinch sea salt
- 1 ½ cups croutons
- 1 large egg
- 1 (1 pound) skinless salmon fillet, cut into 1 ½-inch chunk
- cooking spray

Directions:
1. Mix chipotle powder, maple syrup, and salt in a saucepan and cook on a simmer for 5 minutes.
2. Crush the croutons in a food processor and transfer to a bowl.
3. Beat egg in another shallow bowl.
4. Season the salmon chunks with sea salt.
5. Dip the salmon in the egg, then coat with breadcrumbs.
6. Divide the coated salmon chunks in the two crisper plates.
7. Return the crisper plate to the Ninja Foodi Dual Zone Air Fryer.
8. Select the Air Fry mode for Zone 1 and set the temperature to 390 degrees F and the time to 10 minutes.
9. Press the "MATCH" button to copy the settings for Zone 2.
10. Initiate cooking by pressing the START/STOP button.
11. Flip the chunks once cooked halfway through, then resume cooking.
12. Pour the maple syrup on top and serve warm.
Nutrition Info:
- (Per serving) Calories 275 | Fat 1.4g |Sodium 582mg | Carbs 31.5g | Fiber 1.1g | Sugar 0.1g | Protein 29.8g

Tilapia With Mojo And Crispy Plantains

Servings:4
Cooking Time: 30 Minutes
Ingredients:
- FOR THE TILAPIA
- 4 tilapia fillets (6 ounces each)
- 2 tablespoons all-purpose flour
- Nonstick cooking spray
- ¼ cup freshly squeezed orange juice
- 3 tablespoons fresh lime juice
- 2 tablespoons olive oil
- 1 tablespoon minced garlic
- ½ teaspoon ground cumin
- ¼ teaspoon kosher salt
- FOR THE PLANTAINS
- 1 large green plantain
- 2 cups cold water
- 2 teaspoons kosher salt
- Nonstick cooking spray

Directions:
1. To prep the tilapia: Dust both sides of the tilapia fillets with the flour, then spritz with cooking spray.
2. In a small bowl, whisk together the orange juice, lime juice, oil, garlic, cumin, and salt. Set the mojo sauce aside.
3. To prep the plantains: Cut the ends from the plantain, then remove and discard the peel. Slice the plantain into 1-inch rounds.
4. In a large bowl, combine the water, salt, and plantains. Let soak for 15 minutes.
5. Drain the plantains and pat them dry with paper towels. Spray with cooking spray.
6. To cook the tilapia and plantains: Install a crisper plate in each of the two baskets. Place the tilapia in a single layer in the Zone 1 basket (work in batches if needed) and insert the basket in the unit. Place the plantains in the Zone 2 basket and insert the basket in the unit.
7. Select Zone 1, select AIR FRY, set the temperature to 390°F, and set the timer to 10 minutes.
8. Select Zone 2, select AIR FRY, set the temperature to 390°F, and set the timer to 30 minutes. Select SMART FINISH.
9. Press START/PAUSE to begin cooking.
10. When the Zone 2 timer reads 10 minutes, press START/PAUSE. Remove the basket and use silicone-tipped tongs to transfer the plantains, which should be tender, to a cutting board. Use the bottom of a heavy glass to smash each plantain flat. Spray both sides with cooking spray and place them back in the basket. Reinsert the basket and press START/PAUSE to resume cooking.
11. When the Zone 1 timer reads 5 minutes, press START/PAUSE. Remove the basket. Spoon half of the mojo sauce over the tilapia. Reinsert the basket and press START/PAUSE to resume cooking.
12. When cooking is complete, the fish should be cooked through and the plantains crispy. Serve the tilapia and plantains with the remaining mojo sauce for dipping.
Nutrition Info:

- (Per serving) Calories: 380; Total fat: 21g; Saturated fat: 2g; Carbohydrates: 20g; Fiber: 1g; Protein: 35g; Sodium: 217mg

Lemon Pepper Salmon With Asparagus

Servings: 2
Cooking Time: 18
Ingredients:
- 1 cup of green asparagus
- 2 tablespoons of butter
- 2 fillets of salmon, 8 ounces each
- Salt and black pepper, to taste
- 1 teaspoon of lemon juice
- ½ teaspoon of lemon zest
- oil spray, for greasing

Directions:
1. Rinse and trim the asparagus.
2. Rinse and pat dry the salmon fillets.
3. Take a bowl and mix lemon juice, lemon zest, salt, and black pepper.
4. Brush the fish fillet with the rub and place it in the zone 1 basket.
5. Place asparagus in zone 2 basket.
6. Spray the asparagus with oil spray.
7. Set zone 1 to AIRFRY mode for 18 minutes at 390 degrees F.
8. Set the zone 2 to 5 minutes at 390 degrees F, at air fry mode.
9. Hit the smart finish button to finish at the same time.
10. Once done, serve and enjoy.

Nutrition Info:
- (Per serving) Calories 482| Fat 28g| Sodium 209 mg | Carbs 2.8g | Fiber 1.5 g | Sugar 1.4 g | Protein 56.3g

Shrimp With Lemon And Pepper

Servings: 4
Cooking Time: 8 Minutes
Ingredients:
- 455g raw shrimp, peeled and deveined
- 118ml olive oil
- 2 tablespoons lemon juice
- 1 teaspoon black pepper
- ½ teaspoon salt

Directions:
1. Toss shrimp with black pepper, salt, lemon juice and oil in a bowl.
2. Divide the shrimp into the Ninja Foodi 2 Baskets Air Fryer baskets.
3. Return the air fryer basket 1 to Zone 1, and basket 2 to Zone 2 of the Ninja Foodi 2-Basket Air Fryer.
4. Choose the "Air Fry" mode for Zone 1 at 350 degrees F and 8 minutes of cooking time.
5. Select the "MATCH COOK" option to copy the settings for Zone 2.
6. Initiate cooking by pressing the START/PAUSE BUTTON.
7. Serve warm.

Nutrition Info:
- (Per serving) Calories 257 | Fat 10.4g |Sodium 431mg | Carbs 20g | Fiber 0g | Sugar 1.6g | Protein 21g

Flavorful Salmon With Green Beans

Servings: 4
Cooking Time: 10 Minutes
Ingredients:
- 4 ounces green beans
- 1 tablespoon canola oil
- 4 (6-ounce) salmon fillets
- 1/3 cup prepared sesame-ginger sauce
- Kosher salt, to taste
- Black pepper, to taste

Directions:
1. Toss the green beans with a teaspoon each of salt and pepper in a large bowl.
2. Place a crisper plate in each drawer. Place the green beans in the zone 1 drawer and insert it into the unit. Place the salmon into the zone 2 drawer and place it into the unit.
3. Select zone 1, then AIR FRY, and set the temperature to 390 degrees F/ 200 degrees C with a 10-minute timer.
4. Select zone 2, then AIR FRY, and set the temperature to 390 degrees F/ 200 degrees C with a 15-minute timer. Select SYNC. To begin cooking, press the START/STOP button.
5. Press START/STOP to pause the unit when the zone 2 timer reaches 9 minutes. Remove the salmon from the drawer and toss it in the sesame-ginger sauce. To resume cooking, replace the drawer in the device and press START/STOP.
6. When cooking is complete, serve the salmon and green beans immediately.

Nutrition Info:
- (Per serving) Calories 305 | Fat 16g | Sodium 535mg | Carbs 8.7g | Fiber 1g | Sugar 6.4g | Protein 34.9g

Scallops With Greens

Servings: 8
Cooking Time: 13 Minutes.
Ingredients:
- ¾ cup heavy whipping cream
- 1 tablespoon tomato paste
- 1 tablespoon chopped fresh basil
- 1 teaspoon garlic, minced
- ½ teaspoons salt
- ½ teaspoons pepper
- 12 ounces frozen spinach thawed
- 8 jumbo sea scallops

- Vegetable oil to spray

Directions:
1. Season the scallops with vegetable oil, salt, and pepper in a bowl
2. Mix cream with spinach, basil, garlic, salt, pepper, and tomato paste in a bowl.
3. Pour this mixture over the scallops and mix gently.
4. Divide the scallops in the Air Fryers Baskets without using the crisper plate.
5. Return the crisper plate to the Ninja Foodi Dual Zone Air Fryer.
6. Choose the Air Fry mode for Zone 1 and set the temperature to 390 degrees F and the time to 13 minutes.
7. Select the "MATCH" button to copy the settings for Zone 2.
8. Initiate cooking by pressing the START/STOP button.
9. Serve right away

Nutrition Info:
- (Per serving) Calories 266 | Fat 6.3g |Sodium 193mg | Carbs 39.1g | Fiber 7.2g | Sugar 5.2g | Protein 14.8g

Herb Tuna Patties

Servings: 10
Cooking Time: 12 Minutes

Ingredients:
- 2 eggs
- 425g can tuna, drained & diced
- ½ tsp garlic powder
- ½ small onion, minced
- 1 celery stalk, chopped
- 42g parmesan cheese, grated
- 50g breadcrumbs
- ½ tsp dried oregano
- ½ tsp dried basil
- ½ tsp dried thyme
- 15ml lemon juice
- 1 lemon zest
- Pepper
- Salt

Directions:
1. In a bowl, mix tuna with remaining ingredients until well combined.
2. Insert a crisper plate in the Ninja Foodi air fryer baskets.
3. Make patties from the tuna mixture and place them in both baskets.
4. Select zone 1, then select "bake" mode and set the temperature to 380 degrees F for 12 minutes. Press "match" to match zone 2 settings to zone 1. Press "start/stop" to begin. Turn halfway through.

Nutrition Info:
- (Per serving) Calories 86 | Fat 1.5g |Sodium 90mg | Carbs 4.5g | Fiber 0.4g | Sugar 0.6g | Protein 12.8g

Honey Teriyaki Tilapia

Servings: 4
Cooking Time: 10 Minutes

Ingredients:
- 8 tablespoons low-sodium teriyaki sauce
- 3 tablespoons honey
- 2 garlic cloves, minced
- 2 tablespoons extra virgin olive oil
- 3 pieces tilapia (each cut into 2 pieces)

Directions:
1. Combine all the first 4 ingredients to make the marinade.
2. Pour the marinade over the tilapia and let it sit for 20 minutes.
3. Place a crisper plate in each drawer. Place the tilapia in the drawers. Insert the drawers into the unit.
4. Select zone 1, then AIR FRY, then set the temperature to 360 degrees F/ 180 degrees C with a 10-minute timer. To match zone 2 settings to zone 1, choose MATCH. To begin, select START/STOP.
5. Remove the tilapia from the drawers after the timer has finished.

Nutrition Info:
- (Per serving) Calories 350 | Fat 16.4g | Sodium 706mg | Carbs 19.3g | Fiber 0.1g | Sugar 19g | Protein 29.3g

Bang Bang Shrimp

Servings: 4
Cooking Time: 20 Minutes

Ingredients:
- For the shrimp:
- 1 cup corn starch
- Salt and pepper, to taste
- 2 pounds shrimp, peeled and deveined
- ½ to 1 cup buttermilk
- Cooking oil spray
- 1 large egg whisked with 1 teaspoon water
- For the sauce:
- 1/3 cup sweet Thai chili sauce
- ¼ cup sour cream
- ¼ cup mayonnaise
- 2 tablespoons buttermilk
- 1 tablespoon sriracha, or to taste
- Pinch dried dill weed

Directions:
1. Season the corn starch with salt and pepper in a wide, shallow bowl.
2. In a large mixing bowl, toss the shrimp in the buttermilk to coat them.
3. Dredge the shrimp in the seasoned corn starch.
4. Brush with the egg wash after spraying with cooking oil.

5. Place a crisper plate in each drawer. Place the shrimp in a single layer in each. You may need to cook in batches.
6. Select zone 1, then AIR FRY, then set the temperature to 360 degrees F/ 180 degrees C with a 5-minute timer. To match zone 2 settings to zone 1, choose MATCH. To begin, select START/STOP.
7. Meanwhile, combine all the sauce ingredients together in a bowl.
8. Remove the shrimp when the cooking time is over.

Nutrition Info:
- (Per serving) Calories 415 | Fat 15g | Sodium 1875mg | Carbs 28g | Fiber 1g | Sugar 5g | Protein 38g

Garlic Butter Salmon

Servings: 4
Cooking Time: 10 Minutes

Ingredients:
- 4 (6-ounce) boneless, skin-on salmon fillets (preferably wild-caught)
- 4 tablespoons butter, melted
- 2 teaspoons garlic, minced
- 2 teaspoons fresh Italian parsley, chopped (or ¼ teaspoon dried)
- Salt and pepper to taste

Directions:
1. Season the fresh salmon with salt and pepper.
2. Mix together the melted butter, garlic, and parsley in a bowl.
3. Baste the salmon fillets with the garlic butter mixture.
4. Place a crisper plate in each drawer. Put 2 fillets in each drawer. Put the drawers inside the unit.
5. Select zone 1, then AIR FRY, then set the temperature to 360 degrees F/ 180 degrees C with a 10-minute timer. To match zone 2 settings to zone 1, choose MATCH. To begin, select START/STOP.
6. Remove the salmon from the drawers after the timer has finished.

Nutrition Info:
- (Per serving) Calories 338 | Fat 26g | Sodium 309mg | Carbs 1g | Fiber 0g | Sugar 0g | Protein 25g

Salmon With Coconut

Servings: 2
Cooking Time: 15

Ingredients:
- Oil spray, for greasing
- 2 salmon fillets, 6ounces each
- Salt and ground black pepper, to taste
- 1 tablespoon butter, for frying
- 1 tablespoon red curry paste
- 1 cup of coconut cream
- 2 tablespoons fresh cilantro, chopped
- 1 cup of cauliflower florets
- ½ cup Parmesan cheese, hard

Directions:
1. Take a bowl and mix salt, black pepper, butter, red curry paste, coconut cream in a bowl and marinate the salmon in it.
2. Oil sprays the cauliflower florets and then seasons it with salt and freshly ground black pepper.
3. Put the florets in the zone 1 basket.
4. Layer the parchment paper over the zone 2 baskets, and then place the salmon fillet on it.
5. Set the zone 2 basket to AIR FRY mod at 15 minutes for 400 degrees F
6. Hit the smart finish button to finish it at the same time.
7. Once the time for cooking is over, serve the salmon with cauliflower floret with Parmesan cheese drizzle on top.

Nutrition Info:
- (Per serving) Calories 774 | Fat 59g| Sodium 1223mg | Carbs 12.2g | Fiber 3.9g | Sugar 5.9 g | Protein 53.5 g

Frozen Breaded Fish Fillet

Servings: 2
Cooking Time: 12

Ingredients:
- 4 Frozen Breaded Fish Fillet
- Oil spray, for greasing
- 1 cup mayonnaise

Directions:
1. Take the frozen fish fillets out of the bag and place them in both baskets of the air fryer.
2. Lightly grease it with oil spray.
3. Set the Zone 1 basket to 380 degrees F fo12 minutes.
4. Select the MATCH button for the zone 2 basket.
5. hit the start button to start cooking.
6. Once the cooking is done, serve the fish hot with mayonnaise.

Nutrition Info:
- (Per serving) Calories 921| Fat 61.5g| Sodium 1575mg | Carbs 69g | Fiber 2g | Sugar 9.5g | Protein 29.1g

Stuffed Mushrooms With Crab

Servings: 4
Cooking Time: 18 Minutes

Ingredients:
- 907g baby bella mushrooms
- cooking spray
- 2 teaspoons tony chachere's salt blend
- ¼ red onion, diced
- 2 celery ribs, diced
- 227g lump crab
- ½ cup seasoned bread crumbs
- 1 large egg
- ½ cup parmesan cheese, shredded
- 1 teaspoon oregano

- 1 teaspoon hot sauce

Directions:
1. Mix all the ingredients except the mushrooms in a bowl.
2. Divide the crab filling into the mushroom caps.
3. Place the caps in the air fryer baskets.
4. Return the air fryer basket 1 to Zone 1, and basket 2 to Zone 2 of the Ninja Foodi 2-Basket Air Fryer.
5. Choose the "Air Fry" mode for Zone 1 at 400 degrees F and 18 minutes of cooking time.
6. Select the "MATCH COOK" option to copy the settings for Zone 2.
7. Initiate cooking by pressing the START/PAUSE BUTTON.
8. Serve warm.

Nutrition Info:
- (Per serving) Calories 399 | Fat 16g |Sodium 537mg | Carbs 28g | Fiber 3g | Sugar 10g | Protein 35g

Smoked Salmon

Servings:4
Cooking Time:12

Ingredients:
- 2 pounds of salmon fillets, smoked
- 6 ounces cream cheese
- 4 tablespoons mayonnaise
- 2 teaspoons of chives, fresh
- 1 teaspoon of lemon zest
- Salt and freshly ground black pepper, to taste
- 2 tablespoons of butter

Directions:
1. Cut the salmon into very small and uniform bite-size pieces.
2. Mix cream cheese, chives, mayonnaise, black pepper, and lemon zest, in a small mixing bowl.
3. Let it sit aside for further use.
4. Coat the salmon pieces with salt and butter.
5. Divide the bite-size pieces into both zones of the air fryer.
6. Set it on AIRFRY mode at 400 degrees F for 12 minutes.
7. Select MATCH for zone 2 basket.
8. Hit start, so the cooking start.
9. Once the salmon is done, top it with a bowl creamy mixture and serve.
10. Enjoy hot.

Nutrition Info:
- (Per serving) Calories 557| Fat 15.7 g| Sodium 371mg | Carbs 4.8 g | Fiber 0g | Sugar 1.1g | Protein 48 g

Herb Lemon Mussels

Servings: 6
Cooking Time: 10 Minutes

Ingredients:
- 1kg mussels, steamed & half shell
- 1 tbsp thyme, chopped
- 1 tbsp parsley, chopped
- 1 tsp dried parsley
- 1 tsp garlic, minced
- 60ml olive oil
- 45ml lemon juice
- Pepper
- Salt

Directions:
1. In a bowl, mix mussels with the remaining ingredients.
2. Insert a crisper plate in the Ninja Foodi air fryer baskets.
3. Add the mussels to both baskets.
4. Select zone 1 then select "air fry" mode and set the temperature to 360 degrees F for 10 minutes. Press "match" to match zone 2 settings to zone 1. Press "start/stop" to begin.

Nutrition Info:
- (Per serving) Calories 206 | Fat 11.9g |Sodium 462mg | Carbs 6.3g | Fiber 0.3g | Sugar 0.2g | Protein 18.2g

Shrimp Po'boys With Sweet Potato Fries

Servings:4
Cooking Time: 30 Minutes

Ingredients:
- FOR THE SHRIMP PO'BOYS
- ½ cup buttermilk
- 1 tablespoon Louisiana-style hot sauce
- ¾ cup all-purpose flour
- ½ cup cornmeal
- ½ teaspoon kosher salt
- ½ teaspoon paprika
- ½ teaspoon garlic powder
- ½ teaspoon freshly ground black pepper
- 1 pound peeled medium shrimp, thawed if frozen
- Nonstock cooking spray
- ½ cup store-bought rémoulade sauce
- 4 French bread rolls, halved lengthwise
- ½ cup shredded lettuce
- 1 tomato, sliced
- FOR THE SWEET POTATO FRIES
- 2 medium sweet potatoes
- 2 teaspoons vegetable oil
- ¼ teaspoon garlic powder
- ¼ teaspoon paprika
- ¼ teaspoon kosher salt

Directions:
1. To prep the shrimp: In a medium bowl, combine the buttermilk and hot sauce. In a shallow bowl, combine the flour, cornmeal, salt, paprika, garlic powder, and black pepper.

2. Add the shrimp to the buttermilk and stir to coat. Remove the shrimp, letting the excess buttermilk drip off, then add to the cornmeal mixture to coat.
3. Spritz the breaded shrimp with cooking spray, then let sit for 10 minutes.
4. To prep the sweet potatoes: Peel the sweet potatoes and cut them lengthwise into ¼-inch-thick sticks (like shoestring fries).
5. In a large bowl, combine the sweet potatoes, oil, garlic powder, paprika, and salt. Toss to coat.
6. To cook the shrimp and fries: Install a crisper plate in each of the two baskets. Place the shrimp in the Zone 1 basket and insert the basket in the unit. Place the sweet potatoes in a single layer in the Zone 2 basket and insert the basket in the unit.
7. Select Zone 1, select AIR FRY, set the temperature to 390°F, and set the timer to 13 minutes.
8. Select Zone 2, select AIR FRY, set the temperature to 400°F, and set the timer to 30 minutes. Select SMART FINISH.
9. Press START/PAUSE to begin cooking.
10. When cooking is complete, the shrimp should be golden and cooked through and the sweet potato fries crisp.
11. Spread the rémoulade on the cut sides of the rolls. Divide the lettuce and tomato among the rolls, then top with the fried shrimp. Serve with the sweet potato fries on the side.

Nutrition Info:
- (Per serving) Calories: 669; Total fat: 22g; Saturated fat: 2g; Carbohydrates: 86g; Fiber: 3.5g; Protein: 33g; Sodium: 1,020mg

Crusted Cod

Servings: 4
Cooking Time: 13 Minutes.

Ingredients:
- 2 lbs. cod fillets
- Salt, to taste
- Freshly black pepper, to taste
- ½ cup all-purpose flour
- 1 large egg, beaten
- 2 cups panko bread crumbs
- 1 teaspoon Old Bay seasoning
- Lemon wedges, for serving
- Tartar sauce, for serving

Directions:
1. Rub the fish with salt and black pepper.
2. Add flour in one shallow bowl, beat eggs in another bowl, and mix panko with Old Bay in a shallow bowl.
3. First coat the fish with flour, then dip it in the eggs and finally coat it with the panko mixture.
4. Place half of the seasoned codfish in each crisper plate.
5. Return the crisper plates to the Ninja Foodi Dual Zone Air Fryer.
6. Choose the Air Fry mode for Zone 1 and set the temperature to 390 degrees F and the time to 13 minutes.
7. Select the "MATCH" button to copy the settings for Zone 2.
8. Initiate cooking by pressing the START/STOP button.
9. Flip the fish once cooked halfway, then resume cooking.
10. Serve warm and fresh with tartar sauce and lemon wedges.

Nutrition Info:
- (Per serving) Calories 155 | Fat 4.2g |Sodium 963mg | Carbs 21.5g | Fiber 0.8g | Sugar 5.7g | Protein 8.1g

Beer Battered Fish Fillet

Servings:2
Cooking Time:14

Ingredients:
- 1 cup all-purpose flour
- 4 tablespoons cornstarch
- 1 teaspoon baking soda
- 8 ounces beer
- 2 egg beaten
- ½ cup all-purpose flour
- 1 teaspoon smoked paprika
- 1 teaspoon salt
- 1/4 teaspoon freshly ground black pepper
- ¼ teaspoon of cayenne pepper
- 2 cod fillets, 1½-inches thick, cut into 4 pieces
- Oil spray, for greasing

Directions:
1. Take a large bowl and combine flour, baking soda, corn starch, and salt
2. In a separate bowl beat eggs along with the beer.
3. In a shallow dish mix paprika, salt, pepper, and cayenne pepper.
4. Dry the codfish fillets with a paper towel.
5. Dip the fish into the eggs and coat it with seasoned flour.
6. Then dip it in the seasoning.
7. Grease the fillet with oil spray.
8. Divide the fillet between both zones.
9. Set zone 1 to AIR FRY mode at 400 degrees F for 14 minutes.
10. Select MACTH button for zone 2 basket.
11. Press start and let the AIR fry do its magic.
12. Once cooking is done, serve the fish.
13. Enjoy it hot.

Nutrition Info:
- (Per serving) Calories 1691| Fat 6.1g| Sodium 3976mg | Carbs105.1 g | Fiber 3.4g | Sugar15.6 g | Protein 270g

Furikake Salmon

Servings: 4
Cooking Time: 10 Minutes
Ingredients:
- ½ cup mayonnaise
- 1 tablespoon shoyu
- 455g salmon fillet
- Salt and black pepper to taste
- 2 tablespoons furikake

Directions:
1. Mix shoyu with mayonnaise in a small bowl.
2. Rub the salmon with black pepper and salt.
3. Place the salmon pieces in the air fryer baskets.
4. Top them with the mayo mixture.
5. Return the air fryer basket 1 to Zone 1, and basket 2 to Zone 2 of the Ninja Foodi 2-Basket Air Fryer.
6. Choose the "Air Fry" mode for Zone 1 at 400 degrees F and 10 minutes of cooking time.
7. Select the "MATCH COOK" option to copy the settings for Zone 2.
8. Initiate cooking by pressing the START/PAUSE BUTTON.
9. Serve warm.

Nutrition Info:
- (Per serving) Calories 297 | Fat 1g |Sodium 291mg | Carbs 35g | Fiber 1g | Sugar 9g | Protein 29g

Fish Tacos

Servings: 5
Cooking Time: 30 Minutes
Ingredients:
- 1 pound firm white fish such as cod, haddock, pollock, halibut, or walleye
- ¾ cup gluten-free flour blend
- 3 eggs
- 1 cup gluten-free panko breadcrumbs
- 1 teaspoon garlic powder
- 1 teaspoon onion powder
- 1 teaspoon cumin
- 1 teaspoon lemon pepper
- 1 teaspoon red chili flakes
- 1 teaspoon kosher salt, divided
- 1 teaspoon pepper, divided
- Cooking oil spray
- 1 package corn tortillas
- Toppings such as tomatoes, avocado, cabbage, radishes, jalapenos, salsa, or hot sauce (optional)

Directions:
1. Dry the fish with paper towels. (Make sure to thaw the fish if it's frozen.) Depending on the size of the fillets, cut the fish in half or thirds.
2. On both sides of the fish pieces, liberally season with salt and pepper.
3. Put the flour in a dish.
4. In a separate bowl, crack the eggs and whisk them together until well blended.
5. Put the panko breadcrumbs in another bowl. Add the garlic powder, onion powder, cumin, lemon pepper, and red chili flakes. Add salt and pepper to taste. Stir until everything is well blended.
6. Each piece of fish should be dipped in the flour, then the eggs, and finally in the breadcrumb mixture. Make sure that each piece is completely coated.
7. Put a crisper plate in each drawer. Arrange the fish pieces in a single layer in each drawer. Insert the drawers into the unit.
8. Select zone 1, then AIR FRY, then set the temperature to 360 degrees F/ 180 degrees C with a 20-minute timer. To match zone 2 settings to zone 1, choose MATCH. To begin, select START/STOP.
9. Remove the fish from the drawers after the timer has finished. Place the crispy fish on warmed tortillas.

Nutrition Info:
- (Per serving) Calories 534 | Fat 18g | Sodium 679mg | Carbs 63g | Fiber 8g | Sugar 3g | Protein 27g

Chili Lime Tilapia

Servings: 4
Cooking Time: 10 Minutes
Ingredients:
- 340g tilapia fillets
- 2 teaspoons chili powder
- 1 teaspoon cumin
- 1 teaspoon garlic powder
- ½ teaspoon oregano
- ½ teaspoon sea salt
- ¼ teaspoon black pepper
- Lime zest from 1 lime
- Juice of ½ lime

Directions:
1. Mix chili powder and other spices with lime juice and zest in a bowl.
2. Rub this spice mixture over the tilapia fillets.
3. Place two fillets in each air basket.
4. Return the air fryer basket to the Ninja Foodi 2 Baskets Air Fryer.
5. Choose the "Air Fry" mode for Zone 1 at 400 degrees F and 10 minutes of cooking time.
6. Select the "MATCH COOK" option to copy the settings for Zone 2.
7. Initiate cooking by pressing the START/PAUSE BUTTON.
8. Flip the tilapia fillets once cooked halfway through.
9. Serve warm.

Nutrition Info:
- (Per serving) Calories 275 | Fat 1.4g |Sodium 582mg | Carbs 31.5g | Fiber 1.1g | Sugar 0.1g | Protein 29.8g

Vegetables And Sides Recipes

Air-fried Tofu Cutlets With Cacio E Pepe Brussels Sprouts

Servings: 4
Cooking Time: 25 Minutes
Ingredients:
- FOR THE TOFU CUTLETS
- 1 (14-ounce) package extra-firm tofu, drained
- 1 cup panko bread crumbs
- ¼ cup grated pecorino romano or Parmesan cheese
- 1 teaspoon garlic powder
- 1 teaspoon onion powder
- ¼ teaspoon kosher salt
- 1 tablespoon vegetable oil
- 4 lemon wedges, for serving
- FOR THE BRUSSELS SPROUTS
- 1 pound Brussels sprouts, trimmed
- 1 tablespoon vegetable oil
- 2 tablespoons grated pecorino romano or Parmesan cheese
- ½ teaspoon freshly ground black pepper, plus more to taste
- ¼ teaspoon kosher salt

Directions:
1. To prep the tofu: Cut the tofu horizontally into 4 slabs.
2. In a shallow bowl, mix together the panko, cheese, garlic powder, onion powder, and salt. Press both sides of each tofu slab into the panko mixture. Drizzle both sides with the oil.
3. To prep the Brussels sprouts: Cut the Brussels sprouts in half through the root end.
4. In a large bowl, combine the Brussels sprouts and olive oil. Mix to coat.
5. To cook the tofu cutlets and Brussels sprouts: Install a crisper plate in each of the two baskets. Place the tofu cutlets in a single layer in the Zone 1 basket and insert the basket in the unit. Place the Brussels sprouts in the Zone 2 basket and insert the basket in the unit.
6. Select Zone 1, select AIR FRY, set the temperature to 400°F, and set the timer to 20 minutes.
7. Select Zone 2, select ROAST, set the temperature to 400°F, and set the timer to 25 minutes. Select SMART FINISH.
8. Press START/PAUSE to begin cooking.
9. When both timers read 5 minutes, press START/PAUSE. Remove the Zone 1 basket and use a pair of silicone-tipped tongs to flip the tofu cutlets, then reinsert the basket in the unit. Remove the Zone 2 basket and sprinkle the cheese and black pepper over the Brussels sprouts. Reinsert the basket and press START/PAUSE to resume cooking.
10. When cooking is complete, the tofu should be crisp and the Brussels sprouts tender and beginning to brown.
11. Squeeze the lemon wedges over the tofu cutlets. Stir the Brussels sprouts, then season with the salt and additional black pepper to taste.

Nutrition Info:
- (Per serving) Calories: 319; Total fat: 15g; Saturated fat: 3.5g; Carbohydrates: 27g; Fiber: 6g; Protein: 20g; Sodium: 402mg

Broccoli, Squash, & Pepper

Servings: 4
Cooking Time: 12 Minutes
Ingredients:
- 175g broccoli florets
- 1 red bell pepper, diced
- 1 tbsp olive oil
- ½ tsp garlic powder
- ¼ onion, sliced
- 1 zucchini, sliced
- 2 yellow squash, sliced
- Pepper
- Salt

Directions:
1. In a bowl, toss veggies with oil, garlic powder, pepper, and salt.
2. Insert a crisper plate in the Ninja Foodi air fryer baskets.
3. Add the vegetable mixture in both baskets.
4. Select zone 1 then select "air fry" mode and set the temperature to 390 degrees F for 12 minutes. Press "match" to match zone 2 settings to zone 1. Press "start/stop" to begin. Stir halfway through.

Nutrition Info:
- (Per serving) Calories 75 | Fat 3.9g |Sodium 62mg | Carbs 9.6g | Fiber 2.8g | Sugar 4.8g | Protein 2.9g

Jerk Tofu With Roasted Cabbage

Servings: 4
Cooking Time: 20 Minutes
Ingredients:
- FOR THE JERK TOFU
- 1 (14-ounce) package extra-firm tofu, drained
- 1 tablespoon apple cider vinegar
- 1 tablespoon reduced-sodium soy sauce
- 2 tablespoons jerk seasoning
- Juice of 1 lime
- ½ teaspoon kosher salt
- 2 tablespoons olive oil
- FOR THE CABBAGE
- 1 (14-ounce) bag coleslaw mix
- 1 red bell pepper, thinly sliced

- 2 scallions, thinly sliced
- 2 tablespoons water
- 3 garlic cloves, minced
- ¼ teaspoon fresh thyme leaves
- ¼ teaspoon onion powder
- ¼ teaspoon kosher salt
- ¼ teaspoon freshly ground black pepper

Directions:
1. To prep the jerk tofu: Cut the tofu horizontally into 4 slabs.
2. In a shallow dish (big enough to hold the tofu slabs), whisk together the vinegar, soy sauce, jerk seasoning, lime juice, and salt.
3. Place the tofu in the marinade and turn to coat both sides. Cover and marinate for at least 15 minutes (or up to overnight in the refrigerator).
4. To prep the cabbage: In the Zone 2 basket, combine the coleslaw, bell pepper, scallions, water, garlic, thyme, onion powder, salt, and black pepper.
5. To cook the tofu and cabbage: Install a crisper plate in the Zone 1 basket and add the tofu in a single layer. Brush the tofu with the oil and insert the basket in the unit. Insert the Zone 2 basket in the unit.
6. Select Zone 1, select AIR FRY, set the temperature to 390°F, and set the timer to 15 minutes.
7. Select Zone 2, select ROAST, set the temperature to 330°F, and set the timer to 20 minutes. Select SMART FINISH.
8. Press START/PAUSE to begin cooking.
9. When both timers read 5 minutes, press START/PAUSE. Remove the Zone 1 basket and use silicone-tipped tongs to flip the tofu. Reinsert the basket in the unit. Remove the Zone 2 basket and stir the cabbage. Reinsert the basket and press START/PAUSE to resume cooking.
10. When cooking is complete, the tofu will be crispy and browned around the edges and the cabbage soft.
11. Transfer the tofu to four plates and serve with the cabbage on the side.

Nutrition Info:
- (Per serving) Calories: 220; Total fat: 12g; Saturated fat: 1.5g; Carbohydrates: 21g; Fiber: 5g; Protein: 12g; Sodium: 817mg

Green Beans With Baked Potatoes
Servings: 2
Cooking Time: 45
Ingredients:
- 2 cups of green beans
- 2 large potatoes, cubed
- 3 tablespoons of olive oil
- 1 teaspoon of seasoned salt
- ½ teaspoon chili powder
- 1/6 teaspoon garlic powder
- 1/4 teaspoon onion powder

Directions:
1. Take a large bowl and pour olive oil into it.
2. Now add all the seasoning in the olive oil and whisk it well.
3. Toss the green bean in it, then transfer it to zone 1 basket of the air fryer.
4. Now season the potatoes with the seasoning and add them to the zone 2 basket.
5. Now set the zone one basket to AIRFRY mode at 350 degrees F for 18 minutes.
6. Now hit 2 for the second basket and set it to AIR FRY mode at 350 degrees F, for 45 minutes.
7. Once the cooking cycle is complete, take out and serve it by transferring it to the serving plates.

Nutrition Info:
- (Per serving) Calories473 | Fat21.6g | Sodium796 mg | Carbs 66.6g | Fiber12.9 g | Sugar6 g | Protein8.4 g

Rosemary Asparagus & Potatoes
Servings: 6
Cooking Time: 30 Minutes
Ingredients:
- 125g asparagus, trimmed & cut into pieces
- 2 tsp garlic powder
- 2 tbsp rosemary, chopped
- 30ml olive oil
- 679g baby potatoes, quartered
- ½ tsp red pepper flakes
- Pepper
- Salt

Directions:
1. Insert a crisper plate in the Ninja Foodi air fryer baskets.
2. Toss potatoes with 1 tablespoon of oil, pepper, and salt in a bowl until well coated.
3. Add potatoes into in zone 1 basket.
4. Toss asparagus with remaining oil, red pepper flakes, pepper, garlic powder, and rosemary in a mixing bowl.
5. Add asparagus into the zone 2 basket.
6. Select zone 1, then select "air fry" mode and set the temperature to 390 degrees F for 20 minutes. Select zone 2, then select "air fry" mode and set the temperature to 390 degrees F for 10 minutes. Press "match" mode, then press "start/stop" to begin.

Nutrition Info:
- (Per serving) Calories 121 | Fat 5g |Sodium 40mg | Carbs 17.1g | Fiber 4.2g | Sugar 1g | Protein 4g

Stuffed Sweet Potatoes
Servings: 4
Cooking Time: 55 Minutes
Ingredients:
- 2 medium sweet potatoes
- 1 teaspoon olive oil
- 1 cup cooked chopped spinach, drained
- 1 cup shredded cheddar cheese, divided

- 2 cooked bacon strips, crumbled
- 1 green onion, chopped
- ¼ cup fresh cranberries, coarsely chopped
- 1/3 cup chopped pecans, toasted
- 2 tablespoons butter
- ¼ teaspoon kosher salt
- ¼ teaspoon pepper

Directions:
1. Brush the sweet potatoes with the oil.
2. Place a crisper plate in both drawers. Add one sweet potato to each drawer. Place the drawers in the unit.
3. Select zone 1, then AIR FRY, then set the temperature to 360 degrees F/ 180 degrees C with a 40-minute timer. To match zone 2 settings to zone 1, choose MATCH. To begin, select START/STOP.
4. Remove the sweet potatoes from the drawers after the timer has finished. Cut them in half lengthwise. Scoop out the pulp, leaving a ¼-inch thick shell.
5. Put the pulp in a large bowl and stir in the spinach, ¾ cup of cheese, bacon, onion, pecans, cranberries, butter, salt, and pepper.
6. Spoon the mixture into the potato shells, mounding the mixture slightly.
7. Place a crisper plate in each drawer. Put one filled potato into each drawer and insert them into the unit.
8. Select zone 1, then AIR FRY, then set the temperature to 360 degrees F/ 180 degrees C with a 10-minute timer. To match zone 2 settings to zone 1, choose MATCH. To begin, select START/STOP.
9. Sprinkle with the remaining ¼ cup of cheese. Cook using the same settings until the cheese is melted (about 1 to 2 minutes).

Nutrition Info:
- (Per serving) Calories 376 | Fat 25g | Sodium 489mg | Carbs 28g | Fiber 10g | Sugar 5g | Protein 12g

Air Fried Okra

Servings: 2
Cooking Time: 13 Minutes.
Ingredients:
- ½ lb. okra pods sliced
- 1 teaspoon olive oil
- ¼ teaspoon salt
- 1/8 teaspoon black pepper

Directions:
1. Preheat the Ninja Foodi Dual Zone Air Fryer to 350 degrees F.
2. Toss okra with olive oil, salt, and black pepper in a bowl.
3. Spread the okra in a single layer in the two crisper plates.
4. Return the crisper plate to the Ninja Foodi Dual Zone Air Fryer.
5. Choose the Air Fry mode for Zone 1 and set the temperature to 375 degrees F and the time to 13 minutes.
6. Select the "MATCH" button to copy the settings for Zone 2.
7. Initiate cooking by pressing the START/STOP button.
8. Toss the okra once cooked halfway through, and resume cooking.
9. Serve warm.

Nutrition Info:
- (Per serving) Calories 208 | Fat 5g | Sodium 1205mg | Carbs 34.1g | Fiber 7.8g | Sugar 2.5g | Protein 5.9g

Healthy Air Fried Veggies

Servings: 4
Cooking Time: 15 Minutes
Ingredients:
- 52g onion, sliced
- 71g broccoli florets
- 116g radishes, sliced
- 15ml olive oil
- 100g Brussels sprouts, cut in half
- 325g cauliflower florets
- 1 tsp balsamic vinegar
- ½ tsp garlic powder
- Pepper
- Salt

Directions:
1. In a bowl, toss veggies with oil, vinegar, garlic powder, pepper, and salt.
2. Insert a crisper plate in the Ninja Foodi air fryer baskets.
3. Add veggies in both baskets.
4. Select zone 1 then select "air fry" mode and set the temperature to 380 degrees F for 15 minutes. Press "match" to match zone 2 settings to zone 1. Press "start/stop" to begin. Stir halfway through.

Nutrition Info:
- (Per serving) Calories 71 | Fat 3.8g | Sodium 72mg | Carbs 8.8g | Fiber 3.2g | Sugar 3.3g | Protein 2.5g

Spanakopita Rolls With Mediterranean Vegetable Salad

Servings: 4
Cooking Time: 15 Minutes
Ingredients:
- FOR THE SPANAKOPITA ROLLS
- 1 (10-ounce) package chopped frozen spinach, thawed
- 4 ounces feta cheese, crumbled
- 2 large eggs
- 1 teaspoon dried oregano
- ½ teaspoon freshly ground black pepper
- 12 sheets phyllo dough, thawed
- Nonstick cooking spray
- FOR THE ROASTED VEGETABLES
- 1 medium eggplant, diced

- 1 small red onion, cut into 8 wedges
- 1 red bell pepper, sliced
- 2 tablespoons olive oil
- FOR THE SALAD
- 1 (15-ounce) can chickpeas, drained and rinsed
- ¼ cup chopped fresh parsley
- ¼ cup olive oil
- ¼ cup red wine vinegar
- 2 garlic cloves, minced
- ½ teaspoon dried oregano
- ¼ teaspoon kosher salt
- ¼ teaspoon freshly ground black pepper

Directions:
1. To prep the spanakopita rolls: Squeeze as much liquid from the spinach as you can and place the spinach in a large bowl. Add the feta, eggs, oregano, and black pepper. Mix well.
2. Lay one sheet of phyllo on a clean work surface and mist it with cooking spray. Place another sheet of phyllo directly on top of the first sheet and mist it with cooking spray. Repeat with a third sheet.
3. Spoon one-quarter of the spinach mixture along one short side of the phyllo. Fold the long sides in over the spinach, then roll up it like a burrito.
4. Repeat this process with the remaining phyllo sheets and spinach mixture to form 4 rolls.
5. To prep the vegetables: In a large bowl, combine the eggplant, onion, bell pepper, and oil. Mix well.
6. To cook the rolls and vegetables: Install a crisper plate in each of the two baskets. Place the spanakopita rolls seam-side down in the Zone 1 basket, and spritz the rolls with cooking spray. Place the vegetables in the Zone 2 basket and insert both baskets in the unit.
7. Select Zone 1, select AIR FRY, set the temperature to 375°F, and set the timer to 10 minutes.
8. Select Zone 2, select ROAST, set the temperature to 375°F, and set the timer to 15 minutes. Select SMART FINISH.
9. Press START/PAUSE to begin cooking.
10. When the Zone 1 timer reads 3 minutes, press START/PAUSE. Remove the basket and use silicone-tipped tongs or a spatula to flip the spanakopita rolls. Reinsert the basket and press START/PAUSE to resume cooking.
11. When cooking is complete, the rolls should be crisp and golden brown and the vegetables tender.
12. To assemble the salad: Transfer the roasted vegetables to a large bowl. Stir in the chickpeas and parsley.
13. In a small bowl, whisk together the oil, vinegar, garlic, oregano, salt, and black pepper. Pour the dressing over the vegetables and toss to coat. Serve warm.

Nutrition Info:
- (Per serving) Calories: 739; Total fat: 51g; Saturated fat: 8g; Carbohydrates: 67g; Fiber: 11g; Protein: 21g; Sodium: 806mg

Lime Glazed Tofu

Servings: 6
Cooking Time: 14 Minutes.
Ingredients:
- ⅔ cup coconut aminos
- 2 (14-oz) packages extra-firm, water-packed tofu, drained
- 6 tablespoons toasted sesame oil
- ⅔ cup lime juice

Directions:
1. Pat dry the tofu bars and slice into half-inch cubes.
2. Toss all the remaining ingredients in a small bowl.
3. Marinate for 4 hours in the refrigerator. Drain off the excess water.
4. Divide the tofu cubes in the two crisper plates.
5. Return the crisper plates to the Ninja Foodi Dual Zone Air Fryer.
6. Choose the Air Fry mode for Zone 1 and set the temperature to 400 degrees F and the time to 14 minutes.
7. Select the "MATCH" button to copy the settings for Zone 2.
8. Initiate cooking by pressing the START/STOP button.
9. Toss the tofu once cooked halfway through, then resume cooking.
10. Serve warm.

Nutrition Info:
- (Per serving) Calories 284 | Fat 7.9g | Sodium 704mg | Carbs 38.1g | Fiber 1.9g | Sugar 1.9g | Protein 14.8g

Quinoa Patties

Servings: 4
Cooking Time: 32 Minutes.
Ingredients:
- 1 cup quinoa red
- 1½ cups water
- 1 teaspoon salt
- black pepper, ground
- 1½ cups rolled oats
- 3 eggs beaten
- ¼ cup minced white onion
- ½ cup crumbled feta cheese
- ¼ cup chopped fresh chives
- Salt and black pepper, to taste
- Vegetable or canola oil
- 4 hamburger buns
- 4 arugulas
- 4 slices tomato sliced
- Cucumber yogurt dill sauce
- 1 cup cucumber, diced
- 1 cup Greek yogurt
- 2 teaspoons lemon juice
- ¼ teaspoon salt
- Black pepper, ground

- 1 tablespoon chopped fresh dill
- 1 tablespoon olive oil

Directions:
1. Add quinoa to a saucepan filled with cold water, salt, and black pepper, and place it over medium-high heat.
2. Cook the quinoa to a boil, then reduce the heat, cover, and cook for 20 minutes on a simmer.
3. Fluff and mix the cooked quinoa with a fork and remove it from the heat.
4. Spread the quinoa in a baking stay.
5. Mix eggs, oats, onion, herbs, cheese, salt, and black pepper.
6. Stir in quinoa, then mix well. Make 4 patties out of this quinoa cheese mixture.
7. Divide the patties in the two crisper plates and spray them with cooking oil.
8. Return the crisper plates to the Ninja Foodi Dual Zone Air Fryer.
9. Choose the Air Fry mode for Zone 1 and set the temperature to 390 degrees F and the time to 13 minutes.
10. Select the "MATCH" button to copy the settings for Zone 2.
11. Initiate cooking by pressing the START/STOP button.
12. Flip the patties once cooked halfway through, and resume cooking.
13. Meanwhile, prepare the cucumber yogurt dill sauce by mixing all of its ingredients in a mixing bowl.
14. Place each quinoa patty in a burger bun along with arugula leaves.
15. Serve with yogurt dill sauce.

Nutrition Info:
- (Per serving) Calories 231 | Fat 9g |Sodium 271mg | Carbs 32.8g | Fiber 6.4g | Sugar 7g | Protein 6.3g

Veggie Burgers With "fried" Onion Rings

Servings:4
Cooking Time: 25 Minutes
Ingredients:
- FOR THE VEGGIE BURGERS
- 1 (15-ounce) can black beans, drained and rinsed
- ½ cup panko bread crumbs
- 1 large egg
- ¼ cup finely chopped red bell pepper
- ¼ cup frozen corn, thawed
- 1 tablespoon olive oil
- ½ teaspoon garlic powder
- ½ teaspoon ground cumin
- ¼ teaspoon smoked paprika
- Nonstick cooking spray
- 4 hamburger buns
- ¼ cup barbecue sauce, for serving
- FOR THE ONION RINGS
- 1 large sweet onion
- ½ cup all-purpose flour
- 2 large eggs
- 1 cup panko bread crumbs
- ½ teaspoon kosher salt
- Nonstick cooking spray

Directions:
1. To prep the veggie burgers: In a large bowl, mash the beans with a potato masher or a fork. Stir in the panko, egg, bell pepper, corn, oil, garlic powder, cumin, and smoked paprika. Mix well.
2. Shape the mixture into 4 patties. Spritz both sides of each patty with cooking spray.
3. To prep the onion rings: Cut the onion into ½-inch-thick rings.
4. Set up a breading station with three small shallow bowls. Place the flour in the first bowl. In the second bowl, beat the eggs. Place the panko and salt in the third bowl.
5. Bread the onions rings in this order: First, dip them into the flour, coating both sides. Then, dip into the beaten egg. Finally, coat them in the panko. Spritz each with cooking spray.
6. To cook the burgers and onion rings: Install a crisper plate in each of the two baskets. Place 2 veggie burgers in the Zone 1 basket. Place the onion rings in the Zone 2 basket and insert both baskets in the unit.
7. Select Zone 1, select AIR FRY, set the temperature to 390°F, and set the timer to 25 minutes.
8. Select Zone 2, select AIR FRY, set the temperature to 375°F, and set the timer to 10 minutes. Select SMART FINISH.
9. Press START/PAUSE to begin cooking.
10. When the Zone 1 timer reads 10 minutes, press START/PAUSE. Remove the basket and use a silicone spatula to flip the burgers. Reinsert the basket and press START/PAUSE to resume cooking.
11. When the Zone 1 timer reads 10 minutes, press START/PAUSE. Remove the basket and transfer the burgers to a plate. Place the 2 remaining burgers in the basket. Reinsert the basket and press START/PAUSE to resume cooking.
12. When both timers read 5 minutes, press START/PAUSE. Remove the Zone 1 basket and flip the burgers, then reinsert the basket. Remove the Zone 2 basket and shake vigorously to rearrange the onion rings and separate any that have stuck together. Reinsert the basket and press START/PAUSE to resume cooking.
13. When cooking is complete, the veggie burgers should be cooked through and the onion rings golden brown.
14. Place 1 burger on each bun. Top with barbecue sauce and serve with onion rings on the side.

Nutrition Info:
- (Per serving) Calories: 538; Total fat: 16g; Saturated fat: 2g; Carbohydrates: 83g; Fiber: 10g; Protein: 19g; Sodium: 914mg

Acorn Squash Slices

Servings: 6
Cooking Time: 10 Minutes
Ingredients:
- 2 medium acorn squashes
- ⅔ cup packed brown sugar
- ½ cup butter, melted

Directions:
1. Cut the squash in half, remove the seeds and slice into ½ inch slices.
2. Place the squash slices in the air fryer baskets.
3. Drizzle brown sugar and butter over the squash slices.
4. Return the air fryer basket 1 to Zone 1, and basket 2 to Zone 2 of the Ninja Foodi 2-Basket Air Fryer.
5. Choose the "Air Fry" mode for Zone 1 and set the temperature to 350 degrees F and 10 minutes of cooking time.
6. Select the "MATCH COOK" option to copy the settings for Zone 2.
7. Initiate cooking by pressing the START/PAUSE BUTTON.
8. Flip the squash once cooked halfway through.
9. Serve.

Nutrition Info:
- (Per serving) Calories 206 | Fat 3.4g |Sodium 174mg | Carbs 35g | Fiber 9.4g | Sugar 5.9g | Protein 10.6g

Sweet Potatoes & Brussels Sprouts

Servings: 8
Cooking Time: 35 Minutes
Ingredients:
- 340g sweet potatoes, cubed
- 30ml olive oil
- 150g onion, cut into pieces
- 352g Brussels sprouts, halved
- Pepper
- Salt
- For glaze:
- 78ml ketchup
- 115ml balsamic vinegar
- 15g mustard
- 29 ml honey

Directions:
1. In a bowl, toss Brussels sprouts, oil, onion, sweet potatoes, pepper, and salt.
2. Insert a crisper plate in the Ninja Foodi air fryer baskets.
3. Add Brussels sprouts and sweet potato mixture in both baskets.
4. Select zone 1, then select "air fry" mode and set the temperature to 390 degrees F for 25 minutes. Press "match" to match zone 2 settings to zone 1. Press "start/stop" to begin. Stir halfway through.
5. Meanwhile, add vinegar, ketchup, honey, and mustard to a saucepan and cook over medium heat for 5-10 minutes.
6. Toss cooked sweet potatoes and Brussels sprouts with sauce.

Nutrition Info:
- (Per serving) Calories 142 | Fat 4.2g |Sodium 147mg | Carbs 25.2g | Fiber 4g | Sugar 8.8g | Protein 2.9g

Mixed Air Fry Veggies

Servings:4
Cooking Time:25
Ingredients:
- 2 cups of carrots, cubed
- 2 cups of potatoes, cubed
- 2 cups of shallots, cubed
- 2 cups zucchini, diced
- 2 cups yellow squash, cubed
- Salt and black pepper, to taste
- 1 tablespoon of Italian seasoning
- 2 tablespoons of ranch seasoning
- 4 tablespoons of olive oil

Directions:
1. Take a large bowl and add all the veggies to it.
2. Season the veggies with salt, pepper, Italian seasoning, ranch seasoning, and olive oil
3. Toss all the ingredients well.
4. Now divide this between two baskets of the air fryer.
5. Set zone 1 basket to AIRFRY mode at 360 degrees F for 25 minutes.
6. Select the Match button for the zone 2 basket.
7. Once it is cooked and done, serve, and enjoy.

Nutrition Info:
- (Per serving) Calories 275| Fat 15.3g| Sodium129 mg | Carbs 33g | Fiber3.8 g | Sugar5 g | Protein 4.4g

Bacon Wrapped Corn Cob

Servings: 4
Cooking Time: 10 Minutes
Ingredients:
- 4 trimmed corns on the cob
- 8 bacon slices

Directions:
1. Wrap the corn cobs with two bacon slices.
2. Place the wrapped cobs into the Ninja Foodi 2 Baskets Air Fryer baskets.
3. Return the air fryer basket 1 to Zone 1, and basket 2 to Zone 2 of the Ninja Foodi 2-Basket Air Fryer.
4. Choose the "Air Fry" mode for Zone 1 and set the temperature to 355 degrees F and 10 minutes of cooking time.
5. Select the "MATCH COOK" option to copy the settings for Zone 2.
6. Initiate cooking by pressing the START/PAUSE BUTTON.

7. Flip the corn cob once cooked halfway through.
8. Serve warm.

Nutrition Info:
- (Per serving) Calories 350 | Fat 2.6g | Sodium 358mg | Carbs 64.6g | Fiber 14.4g | Sugar 3.3g | Protein 19.9g

Zucchini Cakes

Servings: 6
Cooking Time: 32 Minutes.

Ingredients:
- 2 medium zucchinis, grated
- 1 cup corn kernel
- 1 medium potato cooked
- 2 tablespoons chickpea flour
- 2 garlic minced
- 2 teaspoons olive oil
- Salt and black pepper
- For Serving:
- Yogurt tahini sauce

Directions:
1. Mix grated zucchini with a pinch of salt in a colander and leave them for 15 minutes.
2. Squeeze out their excess water.
3. Mash the cooked potato in a large-sized bowl with a fork.
4. Add zucchini, corn, garlic, chickpea flour, salt, and black pepper to the bowl.
5. Mix these fritters' ingredients together and make 2 tablespoons-sized balls out of this mixture and flatten them lightly.
6. Divide the fritters in the two crisper plates in a single layer and spray them with cooking.
7. Return the crisper plates to the Ninja Foodi Dual Zone Air Fryer.
8. Choose the Air Fry mode for Zone 1 and set the temperature to 390 degrees F and the time to 17 minutes.
9. Select the "MATCH" button to copy the settings for Zone 2.
10. Initiate cooking by pressing the START/STOP button.
11. Flip the fritters once cooked halfway through, then resume cooking.
12. Serve.

Nutrition Info:
- (Per serving) Calories 270 | Fat 14.6g | Sodium 394mg | Carbs 31.3g | Fiber 7.5g | Sugar 9.7g | Protein 6.4g

Green Tomato Stacks

Servings: 6
Cooking Time: 12 Minutes

Ingredients:
- ¼ cup mayonnaise
- ¼ teaspoon lime zest, grated
- 2 tablespoons lime juice
- 1 teaspoon minced fresh thyme
- ½ teaspoon black pepper
- ¼ cup all-purpose flour
- 2 large egg whites, beaten
- ¾ cup cornmeal
- ¼ teaspoon salt
- 2 medium green tomatoes
- 2 medium re tomatoes
- Cooking spray
- 8 slices Canadian bacon, warmed

Directions:
1. Mix mayonnaise with ¼ teaspoon black pepper, thyme, lime juice and zest in a bowl.
2. Spread flour in one bowl, beat egg whites in another bowl and mix cornmeal with ¼ teaspoon black pepper and salt in a third bowl.
3. Cut the tomatoes into 4 slices and coat each with the flour then dip in the egg whites.
4. Coat the tomatoes slices with the cornmeal mixture.
5. Place the slices in the air fryer baskets.
6. Return the air fryer basket 1 to Zone 1, and basket 2 to Zone 2 of the Ninja Foodi 2-Basket Air Fryer.
7. Choose the "Air Fry" mode for Zone 1 at 390 degrees F and 12 minutes of cooking time.
8. Select the "MATCH COOK" option to copy the settings for Zone 2.
9. Initiate cooking by pressing the START/PAUSE BUTTON.
10. Flip the tomatoes once cooked halfway through.
11. Place the green tomato slices on the working surface.
12. Top them with bacon, and red tomato slice.
13. Serve.

Nutrition Info:
- (Per serving) Calories 113 | Fat 3g | Sodium 152mg | Carbs 20g | Fiber 3g | Sugar 1.1g | Protein 3.5g

Fried Artichoke Hearts

Servings: 6
Cooking Time: 10 Minutes.

Ingredients:
- 3 cans Quartered Artichokes, drained
- ½ cup mayonnaise
- 1 cup panko breadcrumbs
- ⅓ cup grated Parmesan
- salt and black pepper to taste
- Parsley for garnish

Directions:
1. Mix mayonnaise with salt and black pepper and keep the sauce aside.
2. Spread panko breadcrumbs in a bowl.
3. Coat the artichoke pieces with the breadcrumbs.
4. As you coat the artichokes, place them in the two crisper plates in a single layer, then spray them with cooking oil.

5. Return the crisper plates to the Ninja Foodi Dual Zone Air Fryer.
6. Choose the Air Fry mode for Zone 1 and set the temperature to 375 degrees F and the time to 10 minutes.
7. Select the "MATCH" button to copy the settings for Zone 2.
8. Initiate cooking by pressing the START/STOP button.
9. Flip the artichokes once cooked halfway through, then resume cooking.
10. Serve warm with mayo sauce.

Nutrition Info:
- (Per serving) Calories 193 | Fat 1g | Sodium 395mg | Carbs 38.7g | Fiber 1.6g | Sugar 0.9g | Protein 6.6g

Air-fried Radishes

Servings: 6
Cooking Time: 15 Minutes

Ingredients:
- 1020g radishes, quartered
- 3 tablespoons olive oil
- 1 tablespoon fresh oregano, minced
- ¼ teaspoon salt
- ⅛ teaspoon black pepper

Directions:
1. Toss radishes with oil, black pepper, salt and oregano in a bowl.
2. Divide the radishes into the Ninja Foodi 2 Baskets Air Fryer baskets.
3. Return the air fryer basket 1 to Zone 1, and basket 2 to Zone 2 of the Ninja Foodi 2-Basket Air Fryer.
4. Choose the "Air Fry" mode for Zone 1 at 375 degrees F and 15 minutes of cooking time.
5. Select the "MATCH COOK" option to copy the settings for Zone 2.
6. Initiate cooking by pressing the START/PAUSE BUTTON.
7. Toss the radishes once cooked halfway through.
8. Serve.

Nutrition Info:
- (Per serving) Calories 270 | Fat 14.6g | Sodium 394mg | Carbs 31.3g | Fiber 7.5g | Sugar 9.7g | Protein 6.4g

Curly Fries

Servings: 6
Cooking Time: 20 Minutes.

Ingredients:
- 2 spiralized zucchinis
- 1 cup flour
- 2 tablespoons paprika
- 1 teaspoon cayenne pepper
- 1 teaspoon garlic powder
- 1 teaspoon black pepper
- 1 teaspoon salt
- 2 eggs
- Olive oil or cooking spray

Directions:
1. Mix flour with paprika, cayenne pepper, garlic powder, black pepper, and salt in a bowl.
2. Beat eggs in another bowl and dip the zucchini in the eggs.
3. Coat the zucchini with the flour mixture and divide it into two crisper plates.
4. Spray the zucchini with cooking oil.
5. Return the crisper plate to the Ninja Foodi Dual Zone Air Fryer.
6. Choose the Air Fry mode for Zone 1 and set the temperature to 400 degrees F and the time to 20 minutes.
7. Select the "MATCH" button to copy the settings for Zone 2.
8. Initiate cooking by pressing the START/STOP button.
9. Toss the zucchini once cooked halfway through, then resume cooking.
10. Serve warm.

Nutrition Info:
- (Per serving) Calories 212 | Fat 11.8g | Sodium 321mg | Carbs 24.6g | Fiber 4.4g | Sugar 8g | Protein 7.3g

Bacon Potato Patties

Servings: 2
Cooking Time: 15 Minutes

Ingredients:
- 1 egg
- 600g mashed potatoes
- 119g breadcrumbs
- 2 bacon slices, cooked & chopped
- 235g cheddar cheese, shredded
- 15g flour
- Pepper
- Salt

Directions:
1. In a bowl, mix mashed potatoes with remaining ingredients until well combined.
2. Make patties from potato mixture and place on a plate.
3. Place plate in the refrigerator for 10 minutes
4. Insert a crisper plate in the Ninja Foodi air fryer baskets.
5. Place the prepared patties in both baskets.
6. Select zone 1 then select "air fry" mode and set the temperature to 390 degrees F for 15 minutes. Press "match" to match zone 2 settings to zone 1. Press "start/stop" to begin. Turn halfway through.

Nutrition Info:
- (Per serving) Calories 702 | Fat 26.8g | Sodium 1405mg | Carbs 84.8g | Fiber 2.7g | Sugar 3.8g | Protein 30.5g

Garlic-rosemary Brussels Sprouts

Servings: 4
Cooking Time: 8 Minutes
Ingredients:
- 3 tablespoons olive oil
- 2 garlic cloves, minced
- ½ teaspoon salt
- ¼ teaspoon black pepper
- 455g Brussels sprouts, halved
- ½ cup panko bread crumbs
- 1-½ teaspoons rosemary, minced

Directions:
1. Toss the Brussels sprouts with crumbs and the rest of the ingredients in a bowl.
2. Divide the sprouts into the Ninja Foodi 2 Baskets Air Fryer baskets.
3. Return the air fryer basket 1 to Zone 1, and basket 2 to Zone 2 of the Ninja Foodi 2-Basket Air Fryer.
4. Choose the "Air Fry" mode for Zone 1 at 350 degrees F and 8 minutes of cooking time.
5. Select the "MATCH COOK" option to copy the settings for Zone 2.
6. Initiate cooking by pressing the START/PAUSE BUTTON.
7. Toss the Brussels sprouts once cooked halfway through.
8. Serve warm.

Nutrition Info:
- (Per serving) Calories 231 | Fat 9g |Sodium 271mg | Carbs 32.8g | Fiber 6.4g | Sugar 7g | Protein 6.3g

Hasselback Potatoes

Servings: 4
Cooking Time: 15 Minutes.
Ingredients:
- 4 medium Yukon Gold potatoes
- 3 tablespoons melted butter
- 1 tablespoon olive oil
- 3 garlic cloves, crushed
- ½ teaspoon ground paprika
- Salt and black pepper ground, to taste
- 1 tablespoon chopped fresh parsley

Directions:
1. Slice each potato from the top to make ¼-inch slices without cutting its ½-inch bottom, keeping the potato's bottom intact.
2. Mix butter with olive oil, garlic, and paprika in a small bowl.
3. Brush the garlic mixture on top of each potato and add the mixture into the slits.
4. Season them with salt and black pepper.
5. Place 2 seasoned potatoes in each of the crisper plate
6. Return the crisper plate to the Ninja Foodi Dual Zone Air Fryer.
7. Choose the Air Fry mode for Zone 1 and set the temperature to 375 degrees F and the time to 25 minutes.
8. Select the "MATCH" button to copy the settings for Zone 2.
9. Initiate cooking by pressing the START/STOP button.
10. Brushing the potatoes again with butter mixture after 15 minutes, then resume cooking.
11. Garnish with parsley.
12. Serve warm.

Nutrition Info:
- (Per serving) Calories 350 | Fat 2.6g |Sodium 358mg | Carbs 64.6g | Fiber 14.4g | Sugar 3.3g | Protein 19.9g

Buffalo Seitan With Crispy Zucchini Noodles

Servings:4
Cooking Time: 12 Minutes
Ingredients:
- FOR THE BUFFALO SEITAN
- 1 (8-ounce) package precooked seitan strips
- 1 teaspoon garlic powder, divided
- ½ teaspoon onion powder
- ¼ teaspoon smoked paprika
- ¼ cup Louisiana-style hot sauce
- 2 tablespoons vegetable oil
- 1 tablespoon tomato paste
- ¼ teaspoon freshly ground black pepper
- FOR THE ZUCCHINI NOODLES
- 3 large egg whites
- 1¼ cups all-purpose flour
- 1 teaspoon kosher salt, divided
- 12 ounces seltzer water or club soda
- 5 ounces zucchini noodles
- Nonstick cooking spray

Directions:
1. To prep the Buffalo seitan: Season the seitan strips with ½ teaspoon of garlic powder, the onion powder, and smoked paprika.
2. In a large bowl, whisk together the hot sauce, oil, tomato paste, remaining ½ teaspoon of garlic powder, and the black pepper. Set the bowl of Buffalo sauce aside.
3. To prep the zucchini noodles: In a medium bowl, use a handheld mixer to beat the egg whites until stiff peaks form.
4. In a large bowl, combine the flour and ½ teaspoon of salt. Mix in the seltzer to form a thin batter. Fold in the beaten egg whites.
5. Add the zucchini to the batter and gently mix to coat.
6. To cook the seitan and zucchini noodles: Install a crisper plate in each of the two baskets. Place the seitan in the Zone 1 basket and insert the basket in the unit.

Lift the noodles from the batter one at a time, letting the excess drip off, and place them in the Zone 2 basket. Insert the basket in the unit.
7. Select Zone 1, select BAKE, set the temperature to 370°F, and set the timer to 12 minutes.
8. Select Zone 2, select AIR FRY, set the temperature to 400°F, and set the timer to 12 minutes. Select SMART FINISH.
9. Press START/PAUSE to begin cooking.
10. When the Zone 1 timer reads 2 minutes, press START/PAUSE. Remove the basket and transfer the seitan to the bowl of Buffalo sauce. Turn to coat, then return the seitan to the basket. Reinsert the basket and press START/PAUSE to resume cooking.
11. When cooking is complete, the seitan should be warmed through and the zucchini noodles crisp and light golden brown.
12. Sprinkle the zucchini noodles with the remaining ½ teaspoon of salt. If desired, drizzle extra Buffalo sauce over the seitan. Serve hot.

Nutrition Info:
- (Per serving) Calories: 252; Total fat: 15g; Saturated fat: 1g; Carbohydrates: 22g; Fiber: 1.5g; Protein: 13g; Sodium: 740mg

Fried Avocado Tacos

Servings: 4
Cooking Time: 10 Minutes
Ingredients:
- For the sauce:
- 2 cups shredded fresh kale or coleslaw mix
- ¼ cup minced fresh cilantro
- ¼ cup plain Greek yogurt
- 2 tablespoons lime juice
- 1 teaspoon honey
- ¼ teaspoon salt
- ¼ teaspoon ground chipotle pepper
- ¼ teaspoon pepper
- For the tacos:
- 1 large egg, beaten
- ¼ cup cornmeal
- ½ teaspoon salt
- ½ teaspoon garlic powder
- ½ teaspoon ground chipotle pepper
- 2 medium avocados, peeled and sliced
- Cooking spray
- 8 flour tortillas or corn tortillas (6 inches), heated up
- 1 medium tomato, chopped
- Crumbled queso fresco (optional)

Directions:
1. Combine the first 8 ingredients in a bowl. Cover and refrigerate until serving.
2. Place the egg in a shallow bowl. In another shallow bowl, mix the cornmeal, salt, garlic powder, and chipotle pepper.
3. Dip the avocado slices in the egg, then into the cornmeal mixture, gently patting to help adhere.
4. Place a crisper plate in both drawers. Put the avocado slices in the drawers in a single layer. Insert the drawers into the unit.
5. Select zone 1, then AIR FRY, then set the temperature to 360 degrees F/ 180 degrees C with a 6-minute timer. To match zone 2 settings to zone 1, choose MATCH. To begin, select START/STOP.
6. Put the avocado slices, prepared sauce, tomato, and queso fresco in the tortillas and serve.

Nutrition Info:
- (Per serving) Calories 407 | Fat 21g | Sodium 738mg | Carbs 48g | Fiber 4g | Sugar 9g | Protein 9g

Fried Patty Pan Squash

Servings: 6
Cooking Time: 15 Minutes
Ingredients:
- 5 cups small pattypan squash, halved
- 1 tablespoon olive oil
- 2 garlic cloves, minced
- ½ teaspoon salt
- ¼ teaspoon dried oregano
- ¼ teaspoon dried thyme
- ¼ teaspoon pepper
- 1 tablespoon minced parsley

Directions:
1. Rub the squash with oil, garlic and the rest of the ingredients.
2. Spread the squash in the air fryer baskets.
3. Return the air fryer basket 1 to Zone 1, and basket 2 to Zone 2 of the Ninja Foodi 2-Basket Air Fryer.
4. Choose the "Air Fry" mode for Zone 1 at 375 degrees F and 15 minutes of cooking time.
5. Select the "MATCH COOK" option to copy the settings for Zone 2.
6. Initiate cooking by pressing the START/PAUSE BUTTON.
7. Flip the squash once cooked halfway through.
8. Garnish with parsley.
9. Serve warm.

Nutrition Info:
- (Per serving) Calories 208 | Fat 5g |Sodium 1205mg | Carbs 34.1g | Fiber 7.8g | Sugar 2.5g | Protein 5.9g

Delicious Potatoes & Carrots

Servings: 8
Cooking Time: 25 Minutes
Ingredients:
- 453g carrots, sliced
- 2 tsp smoked paprika
- 21g sugar
- 30ml olive oil
- 453g potatoes, diced
- ¼ tsp thyme

- ½ tsp dried oregano
- 1 tsp garlic powder
- Pepper
- Salt

Directions:
1. In a bowl, toss carrots and potatoes with 1 tablespoon of oil.
2. Insert a crisper plate in the Ninja Foodi air fryer baskets.
3. Add carrots and potatoes to both baskets.
4. Select zone 1 then select "air fry" mode and set the temperature to 390 degrees F for 15 minutes. Press "match" to match zone 2 settings to zone 1. Press "start/stop" to begin.
5. In a mixing bowl, add cooked potatoes, carrots, smoked paprika, sugar, oil, thyme, oregano, garlic powder, pepper, and salt and toss well.
6. Return carrot and potato mixture into the air fryer basket and cook for 10 minutes more.

Nutrition Info:
- (Per serving) Calories 101 | Fat 3.6g |Sodium 62mg | Carbs 16.6g | Fiber 3g | Sugar 5.1g | Protein 1.6g

Garlic Potato Wedges In Air Fryer

Servings:2
Cooking Time:23
Ingredients:
- 4 medium potatoes, peeled and cut into wedges
- 4 tablespoons of butter
- 1 teaspoon of chopped cilantro
- 1 cup plain flour
- 1 teaspoon of garlic, minced
- Salt and black pepper, to taste

Directions:
1. Soak the potatoes wedges in cold water for about 30 minutes.
2. Then drain and pat dry with a paper towel.
3. Boil water in a large pot and boil the wedges just for 3 minutes.
4. Then take it out on a paper towel.
5. Now in a bowl mix garlic, melted butter, salt, pepper, cilantro and whisk it well.
6. Add the flour to a separate bowl and add salt and black pepper.
7. Then add water to the flour so it gets runny in texture.
8. Now, coat the potatoes with flour mixture and add it to two foil tins.
9. Put foil tins in both the air fryer basket.
10. Now, set time for zone 1 basket using AIRFRY mode at 390 degrees F for 20 minutes.
11. Select the MATCH button for the zone 2 basket.
12. Once done, serve and enjoy.

Nutrition Info:
- (Per serving) Calories 727| Fat 24.1g| Sodium 191mg | Carbs 115.1g | Fiber 12g | Sugar 5.1g | Protein14 g

Fried Asparagus

Servings: 4
Cooking Time: 6 Minutes
Ingredients:
- ¼ cup mayonnaise
- 4 teaspoons olive oil
- 1½ teaspoons grated lemon zest
- 1 garlic clove, minced
- ½ teaspoon pepper
- ¼ teaspoon seasoned salt
- 1-pound fresh asparagus, trimmed
- 2 tablespoons shredded parmesan cheese
- Lemon wedges (optional)

Directions:
1. In a large bowl, combine the first 6 ingredients.
2. Add the asparagus; toss to coat.
3. Put a crisper plate in both drawers. Put the asparagus in a single layer in each drawer. Top with the parmesan cheese. Place the drawers into the unit.
4. Select zone 1, then AIR FRY, then set the temperature to 375 degrees F/ 190 degrees C with a 6-minute timer. To match zone 2 settings to zone 1, choose MATCH. To begin, select START/STOP.
5. Remove the asparagus from the drawers after the timer has finished.

Nutrition Info:
- (Per serving) Calories 156 | Fat 15g | Sodium 214mg | Carbs 3g | Fiber 1g | Sugar 1g | Protein 2g

Garlic-herb Fried Squash

Servings: 4
Cooking Time: 15 Minutes
Ingredients:
- 5 cups halved small pattypan squash (about 1¼ pounds)
- 1 tablespoon olive oil
- 2 garlic cloves, minced
- ½ teaspoon salt
- ¼ teaspoon dried oregano
- ¼ teaspoon dried thyme
- ¼ teaspoon pepper
- 1 tablespoon minced fresh parsley, for serving

Directions:
1. Place the squash in a large bowl.
2. Mix the oil, garlic, salt, oregano, thyme, and pepper; drizzle over the squash. Toss to coat.
3. Place a crisper plate in both drawers. Put the squash in a single layer in each drawer. Insert the drawers into the unit.
4. Select zone 1, then AIR FRY, then set the temperature to 360 degrees F/ 180 degrees C with a 6-

minute timer. To match zone 2 settings to zone 1, choose MATCH. To begin, select START/STOP.
5. Remove the squash from the drawers after the timer has finished. Sprinkle with the parsley.
Nutrition Info:
- (Per serving) Calories 58 | Fat 3g | Sodium 296mg | Carbs 6g | Fiber 2g | Sugar 3g | Protein 2g

Bbq Corn

Servings: 4
Cooking Time: 10 Minutes
Ingredients:
- 450g can baby corn, drained & rinsed
- 56g BBQ sauce
- ½ tsp Sriracha sauce

Directions:
1. In a bowl, toss the baby corn with sriracha sauce and BBQ sauce until well coated.
2. Insert a crisper plate in the Ninja Foodi air fryer baskets.
3. Add the baby corn to both baskets.
4. Select zone 1, then select "air fry" mode and set the temperature to 390 degrees F for 10 minutes. Press "match" to match zone 2 settings to zone 1. Press "start/stop" to begin. Stir halfway through.

Nutrition Info:
- (Per serving) Calories 46 | Fat 0.1g |Sodium 446mg | Carbs 10.2g | Fiber 2.8g | Sugar 5.9g | Protein 0.9g

Fried Olives

Servings: 6
Cooking Time: 9 Minutes.
Ingredients:
- 2 cups blue cheese stuffed olives, drained
- ½ cup all-purpose flour
- 1 cup panko breadcrumbs
- ½ teaspoon garlic powder
- 1 pinch oregano
- 2 eggs

Directions:
1. Mix flour with oregano and garlic powder in a bowl and beat two eggs in another bowl.
2. Spread panko breadcrumbs in a bowl.
3. Coat all the olives with the flour mixture, dip in the eggs and then coat with the panko breadcrumbs.
4. As you coat the olives, place them in the two crisper plates in a single layer, then spray them with cooking oil.
5. Return the crisper plates to the Ninja Foodi Dual Zone Air Fryer.
6. Choose the Air Fry mode for Zone 1 and set the temperature to 375 degrees F and the time to 9 minutes.
7. Select the "MATCH" button to copy the settings for Zone 2.
8. Initiate cooking by pressing the START/STOP button.

9. Flip the olives once cooked halfway through, then resume cooking.
10. Serve.

Nutrition Info:
- (Per serving) Calories 166 | Fat 3.2g |Sodium 437mg | Carbs 28.8g | Fiber 1.8g | Sugar 2.7g | Protein 5.8g

Mushroom Roll-ups

Servings: 10
Cooking Time: 11 Minutes.
Ingredients:
- 2 tablespoons olive oil
- 227g portobello mushrooms, chopped
- 1 teaspoon dried oregano
- 1 teaspoon dried thyme
- ½ teaspoon crushed red pepper flakes
- ¼ teaspoon salt
- 1 package (227g) cream cheese, softened
- 113g whole-milk ricotta cheese
- 10 (8 inches) flour tortillas
- Cooking spray
- Chutney

Directions:
1. Sauté mushrooms with oil, thyme, salt, pepper flakes, and oregano in a skillet for 4 minutes.
2. Mix cheeses and add sauteed mushrooms the mix well.
3. Divide the mushroom mixture over the tortillas.
4. Roll the tortillas and secure with a toothpick.
5. Place the rolls in the air fryer basket.
6. Return the air fryer basket 1 to Zone 1, and basket 2 to Zone 2 of the Ninja Foodi 2-Basket Air Fryer.
7. Choose the "Air Fry" mode for Zone 1 and set the temperature to 400 degrees F and 11 minutes of cooking time.
8. Select the "MATCH COOK" option to copy the settings for Zone 2.
9. Initiate cooking by pressing the START/PAUSE BUTTON.
10. Flip the rolls once cooked halfway through.
11. Serve warm.

Nutrition Info:
- (Per serving) Calories 288 | Fat 6.9g |Sodium 761mg | Carbs 46g | Fiber 4g | Sugar 12g | Protein 9.6g

Kale And Spinach Chips

Servings:2
Cooking Time:6
Ingredients:
- 2 cups spinach, torn in pieces and stem removed
- 2 cups kale, torn in pieces, stems removed
- 1 tablespoon of olive oil
- Sea salt, to taste
- 1/3 cup Parmesan cheese

Directions:

1. Take a bowl and add spinach to it.
2. Take another bowl and add kale to it.
3. Now, season both of them with olive oil, and sea salt.
4. Add kale to zone 1 basket and spinach to zone 2 basket.
5. Select the zone 1 air fry mode at 350 degrees F for 6 minutes.
6. Set zone 2 to AIR FRY mode at 350 for 5 minutes.
7. Once done, take out the crispy chips and sprinkle Parmesan cheese on top.
8. Serve and Enjoy.

Nutrition Info:
- (Per serving) Calories 166| Fat 11.1g| Sodium 355mg | Carbs 8.1g | Fiber1.7 g | Sugar 0.1g | Protein 8.2g

Potatoes & Beans

Servings: 4
Cooking Time: 25 Minutes

Ingredients:
- 453g potatoes, cut into pieces
- 15ml olive oil
- 1 tsp garlic powder
- 160g green beans, trimmed
- Pepper
- Salt

Directions:
1. In a bowl, toss green beans, garlic powder, potatoes, oil, pepper, and salt.
2. Insert a crisper plate in the Ninja Foodi air fryer baskets.
3. Add green beans and potato mixture to both baskets.
4. Select zone 1 then select "air fry" mode and set the temperature to 380 degrees F for 25 minutes. Press "match" to match zone 2 settings to zone 1. Press "start/stop" to begin. Stir halfway through.

Nutrition Info:
- (Per serving) Calories 128 | Fat 3.7g |Sodium 49mg | Carbs 22.4g | Fiber 4.7g | Sugar 2.3g | Protein 3.1g

Beef, Pork, And Lamb Recipes

Mustard Rubbed Lamb Chops

Servings: 4
Cooking Time: 31 Minutes.

Ingredients:
- 1 teaspoon Dijon mustard
- 1 teaspoon olive oil
- ½ teaspoon soy sauce
- ½ teaspoon garlic, minced
- ½ teaspoon cumin powder
- ½ teaspoon cayenne pepper
- ½ teaspoon Italian spice blend
- ⅛ teaspoon salt
- 4 pieces of lamb chops

Directions:
1. Mix Dijon mustard, soy sauce, olive oil, garlic, cumin powder, cayenne pepper, Italian spice blend, and salt in a medium bowl and mix well.
2. Place lamb chops into a Ziploc bag and pour in the marinade.
3. Press the air out of the bag and seal tightly.
4. Press the marinade around the lamb chops to coat.
5. Keep then in the fridge and marinate for at least 30 minutes, up to overnight.
6. Place 2 chops in each of the crisper plate and spray them with cooking oil.
7. Return the crisper plate to the Ninja Foodi Dual Zone Air Fryer.
8. Select the Roast mode for Zone 1 and set the temperature to 350 degrees F and the time to 27 minutes.
9. Select the "MATCH" button to copy the settings for Zone 2.
10. Initiate cooking by pressing the START/STOP button.
11. Flip the chops once cooked halfway through, and resume cooking.
12. Switch the Roast mode to Max Crisp mode and cook for 5 minutes.
13. Serve warm.

Nutrition Info:
- (Per serving) Calories 264 | Fat 17g |Sodium 129mg | Carbs 0.9g | Fiber 0.3g | Sugar 0g | Protein 27g

Lamb Chops With Dijon Garlic

Servings: 4
Cooking Time: 22 Minutes
Ingredients:
- 2 teaspoons Dijon mustard
- 2 teaspoons olive oil
- 1 teaspoon soy sauce
- 1 teaspoon garlic, minced
- 1 teaspoon cumin powder
- 1 teaspoon cayenne pepper
- 1 teaspoon Italian spice blend (optional)
- ¼ teaspoon salt
- 8 lamb chops

Directions:
1. Combine the Dijon mustard, olive oil, soy sauce, garlic, cumin powder, cayenne pepper, Italian spice blend (optional), and salt in a medium mixing bowl.
2. Put the marinade in a large Ziploc bag. Add the lamb chops. Seal the bag tightly after pressing out the air. Coat the lamb in the marinade by shaking the bag and pressing the chops into the mixture. Place in the fridge for at least 30 minutes, or up to overnight, to marinate.
3. Install a crisper plate in both drawers. Place half the lamb chops in the zone 1 drawer and half in zone 2's, then insert the drawers into the unit.
4. Select zone 1, select AIR FRY, set temperature to 390 degrees F/ 200 degrees C, and set time to 22 minutes. Select MATCH to match zone 2 settings to zone 1. Press the START/STOP button to begin cooking.
5. When the time reaches 11 minutes, press START/STOP to pause the unit. Remove the drawers and flip the lamb chops. Re-insert the drawers into the unit and press START/STOP to resume cooking.
6. Serve and enjoy!

Nutrition Info:
- (Per serving) Calories 343 | Fat 15.1g | Sodium 380mg | Carbs 0.9 g | Fiber 0.3g | Sugar 0.1g | Protein 48.9g

Gochujang Brisket

Servings: 6
Cooking Time: 55 Minutes.
Ingredients:
- ½ tablespoons sweet paprika
- ½ teaspoon toasted sesame oil
- 2 lbs. beef brisket, cut into 4 pieces
- Salt, to taste
- ⅛ cup Gochujang, Korean chili paste
- Black pepper, to taste
- 1 small onion, diced
- 2 garlic cloves, minced
- 1 teaspoon Asian fish sauce
- 1 ½ tablespoons peanut oil, as needed
- ½ tablespoon fresh ginger, grated
- ¼ teaspoon red chili flakes
- ½ cup of water
- 1 tablespoon ketchup
- 1 tablespoon soy sauce

Directions:
1. Thoroughly rub the beef brisket with olive oil, paprika, chili flakes, black pepper, and salt.
2. Cut the brisket in half, then divide the beef in the two crisper plate.
3. Return the crisper plate to the Ninja Foodi Dual Zone Air Fryer.
4. Choose the Air Fry mode for Zone 1 and set the temperature to 390 degrees F and the time to 35 minutes.
5. Select the "MATCH" button to copy the settings for Zone 2.
6. Initiate cooking by pressing the START/STOP button.
7. Flip the brisket halfway through, and resume cooking.
8. Meanwhile, heat oil in a skillet and add ginger, onion, and garlic.
9. Sauté for 5 minutes, then add all the remaining ingredients.
10. Cook the mixture for 15 minutes approximately until well thoroughly mixed.
11. Serve the brisket with this sauce on top.

Nutrition Info:
- (Per serving) Calories 374 | Fat 25g |Sodium 275mg | Carbs 7.3g | Fiber 0g | Sugar 6g | Protein 12.3g

Beef And Bean Taquitos With Mexican Rice

Servings:4
Cooking Time: 15 Minutes
Ingredients:
- FOR THE TAQUITOS
- ½ pound ground beef (85 percent lean)
- 1 tablespoon taco seasoning
- 8 (6-inch) soft white corn tortillas
- Nonstick cooking spray
- ¾ cup canned refried beans
- ½ cup shredded Mexican blend cheese (optional)
- FOR THE MEXICAN RICE
- 1 cup dried instant white rice (not microwavable)
- 1½ cups chicken broth
- ¼ cup jarred salsa
- 2 tablespoons canned tomato sauce
- 1 tablespoon vegetable oil
- ½ teaspoon kosher salt

Directions:
1. To prep the taquitos: In a large bowl, mix the ground beef and taco seasoning until well combined.
2. Mist both sides of each tortilla lightly with cooking spray.

3. To prep the Mexican rice: In the Zone 2 basket, combine the rice, broth, salsa, tomato sauce, oil, and salt. Stir well to ensure all of the rice is submerged in the liquid.
4. To cook the taquitos and rice: Install a crisper plate in the Zone 1 basket. Place the seasoned beef in the basket and insert the basket in the unit. Insert the Zone 2 basket in the unit.
5. Select Zone 1, select AIR FRY, set the temperature to 390°F, and set the time to 15 minutes.
6. Select Zone 2, select BAKE, set the temperature to 350°F, and set the time to 10 minutes. Select SMART FINISH.
7. Press START/PAUSE to begin cooking.
8. When the Zone 1 timer reads 10 minutes, press START/PAUSE. Remove the basket and transfer the beef to a medium bowl. Add the refried beans and cheese (if using) and combine well. Spoon 2 tablespoons of the filling onto each tortilla and roll tightly. Place the taquitos in the Zone 1 basket seam-side down. Reinsert the basket in the unit and press START/PAUSE to resume cooking.
9. When cooking is complete, the taquitos should be crisp and golden brown and the rice cooked through. Serve hot.

Nutrition Info:
- (Per serving) Calories: 431; Total fat: 18g; Saturated fat: 4g; Carbohydrates: 52g; Fiber: 5.5g; Protein: 18g; Sodium: 923mg

Easy Breaded Pork Chops

Servings: 8
Cooking Time: 12 Minutes
Ingredients:
- 1 egg
- 118ml milk
- 8 pork chops
- 1 packet ranch seasoning
- 238g breadcrumbs
- Pepper
- Salt

Directions:
1. In a small bowl, whisk the egg and milk.
2. In a separate shallow dish, mix breadcrumbs, ranch seasoning, pepper, and salt.
3. Dip each pork chop in the egg mixture, then coat with breadcrumbs.
4. Insert a crisper plate in the Ninja Foodi air fryer baskets.
5. Place the coated pork chops in both baskets.
6. Select zone 1, then select air fry mode and set the temperature to 360 degrees F for 12 minutes. Press "match" to match zone 2 settings to zone 1. Press "start/stop" to begin. Turn halfway through.

Nutrition Info:
- (Per serving) Calories 378 | Fat 22.2g |Sodium 298mg | Carbs 20.2g | Fiber 1.2g | Sugar 2.4g | Protein 22.8g

Steak In Air Fry

Servings:1
Cooking Time:20
Ingredients:
- 2 teaspoons of canola oil
- 1 tablespoon of Montreal steaks seasoning
- 1 pound of beef steak

Directions:
1. The first step is to season the steak on both sides with canola oil and then rub a generous amount of steak seasoning all over.
2. We are using the AIR BROIL feature of the ninja air fryer and it works with one basket.
3. Put the steak in the basket and set it to AIR BROIL at 450 degrees F for 20 -22 minutes.
4. After 7 minutes, hit pause and take out the basket to flip the steak, and cover it with foil on top, for the remaining 14 minutes.
5. Once done, serve the medium-rare steak and enjoy it by resting for 10 minutes.
6. Serve by cutting in slices.
7. Enjoy.

Nutrition Info:
- (Per serving) Calories 935| Fat 37.2g| Sodium 1419mg | Carbs 0g | Fiber 0g| Sugar 0g | Protein137.5 g

Garlic Butter Steaks

Servings: 2
Cooking Time: 25 Minutes
Ingredients:
- 2 (6 ounces each) sirloin steaks or ribeyes
- 2 tablespoons unsalted butter
- 1 clove garlic, crushed
- ½ teaspoon dried parsley
- ½ teaspoon dried rosemary
- Salt and pepper, to taste

Directions:
1. Season the steaks with salt and pepper and set them to rest for about 2 hours before cooking.
2. Put the butter in a bowl. Add the garlic, parsley, and rosemary. Allow the butter to soften.
3. Whip together with a fork or spoon once the butter has softened.
4. When you're ready to cook, install a crisper plate in both drawers. Place the sirloin steaks in a single layer in each drawer. Insert the drawers into the unit.
5. Select zone 1, select AIR FRY, set temperature to 360 degrees F/ 180 degrees C, and set time to 10 minutes. Select MATCH to match zone 2 settings to zone 1. Select START/STOP to begin.
6. Once done, serve with the garlic butter.

Nutrition Info:

- (Per serving) Calories 519 | Fat 36g | Sodium 245mg | Carbs 1g | Fiber 0g | Sugar 0g | Protein 46g

Air Fryer Meatloaves

Servings: 4
Cooking Time: 22 Minutes.
Ingredients:
- ⅓ cup milk
- 2 tablespoons basil pesto
- 1 egg, beaten
- 1 garlic clove, minced
- ¼ teaspoons black pepper
- 1 lb. ground beef
- ⅓ cup panko bread crumbs
- 8 pepperoni slices
- ½ cup marinara sauce, warmed
- 1 tablespoon fresh basil, chopped

Directions:
1. Mix pesto, milk, egg, garlic, and black pepper in a medium-sized bowl.
2. Stir in ground beef and bread crumbs, then mix.
3. Make the 4 small-sized loaves with this mixture and top them with 2 pepperoni slices.
4. Press the slices into the meatloaves.
5. Place the meatloaves in the two crisper plates.
6. Return the crisper plate to the Ninja Foodi Dual Zone Air Fryer.
7. Choose the Air Fry mode for Zone 1 and set the temperature to 390 degrees F and the time to 22 minutes.
8. Select the "MATCH" button to copy the settings for Zone 2.
9. Initiate cooking by pressing the START/STOP button.
10. Top them with marinara sauce and basil to serve.
11. Serve warm.

Nutrition Info:
- (Per serving) Calories 316 | Fat 12.2g |Sodium 587mg | Carbs 12.2g | Fiber 1g | Sugar 1.8g | Protein 25.8g

Meatloaf

Servings: 6
Cooking Time: 25 Minutes
Ingredients:
- For the meatloaf:
- 2 pounds ground beef
- 2 eggs, beaten
- 2 cups old-fashioned oats, regular or gluten-free
- ½ cup evaporated milk
- ½ cup chopped onion
- ½ teaspoon garlic salt
- For the sauce:
- 1 cup ketchup
- ¾ cup brown sugar, packed
- ¼ cup chopped onion
- ½ teaspoon liquid smoke
- ¼ teaspoon garlic powder
- Olive oil cooking spray

Directions:
1. In a large bowl, combine all the meatloaf ingredients.
2. Spray 2 sheets of foil with olive oil cooking spray.
3. Form the meatloaf mixture into a loaf shape, cut in half, and place each half on one piece of foil.
4. Roll the foil up a bit on the sides. Allow it to be slightly open.
5. Put all the sauce ingredients in a saucepan and whisk until combined on medium-low heat. This should only take 1–2 minutes
6. Install a crisper plate in both drawers. Place half the meatloaf in the zone 1 drawer and half in zone 2's, then insert the drawers into the unit.
7. Select zone 1, select AIR FRY, set temperature to 390 degrees F/ 200 degrees C, and set time to 25 minutes. Select MATCH to match zone 2 settings to zone 1. Press the START/STOP button to begin cooking.
8. When the time reaches 20 minutes, press START/STOP to pause the unit. Remove the drawers and coat the meatloaf with the sauce using a brush. Re-insert the drawers into the unit and press START/STOP to resume cooking.
9. Carefully remove and serve.

Nutrition Info:
- (Per serving) Calories 727 | Fat 34g | Sodium 688mg | Carbs 57g | Fiber 3g | Sugar 34g | Protein 49g

Turkey And Beef Meatballs

Servings: 6
Cooking Time: 24 Minutes.
Ingredients:
- 1 medium shallot, minced
- 2 tablespoons olive oil
- 3 garlic cloves, minced
- ¼ cup panko crumbs
- 2 tablespoons whole milk
- ⅔ lb. lean ground beef
- ⅓ lb. bulk turkey sausage
- 1 large egg, lightly beaten
- ¼ cup parsley, chopped
- 1 tablespoon fresh thyme, chopped
- 1 tablespoon fresh rosemary, chopped
- 1 tablespoon Dijon mustard
- ½ teaspoon salt

Directions:
1. Preheat your oven to 400 degrees F. Place a medium non-stick pan over medium-high heat.
2. Add oil and shallot, then sauté for 2 minutes.
3. Toss in the garlic and cook for 1 minute.
4. Remove this pan from the heat.
5. Whisk panko with milk in a large bowl and leave it for 5 minutes.

6. Add cooked shallot mixture and mix well.
7. Stir in egg, parsley, turkey sausage, beef, thyme, rosemary, salt, and mustard.
8. Mix well, then divide the mixture into 1 ½-inch balls.
9. Divide these balls into the two crisper plates and spray them with cooking oil.
10. Return the crisper plates to the Ninja Foodi Dual Zone Air Fryer.
11. Choose the Air Fry mode for Zone 1 and set the temperature to 400 degrees F and the time to 21 minutes.
12. Select the "MATCH" button to copy the settings for Zone 2.
13. Initiate cooking by pressing the START/STOP button.
14. Serve warm.

Nutrition Info:
- (Per serving) Calories 551 | Fat 31g |Sodium 1329mg | Carbs 1.5g | Fiber 0.8g | Sugar 0.4g | Protein 64g

Pork With Green Beans And Potatoes

Servings: 4
Cooking Time: 15 Minutes.
Ingredients:
- ¼ cup Dijon mustard
- 2 tablespoons brown sugar
- 1 teaspoon dried parsley flake
- ½ teaspoon dried thyme
- ¼ teaspoons salt
- ¼ teaspoons black pepper
- 1 ¼ lbs. pork tenderloin
- ¾ lb. small potatoes halved
- 1 (12-oz) package green beans, trimmed
- 1 tablespoon olive oil
- Salt and black pepper ground to taste

Directions:
1. Preheat your Air Fryer Machine to 400 degrees F.
2. Add mustard, parsley, brown sugar, salt, black pepper, and thyme in a large bowl, then mix well.
3. Add tenderloin to the spice mixture and coat well.
4. Toss potatoes with olive oil, salt, black pepper, and green beans in another bowl.
5. Place the prepared tenderloin in the crisper plate.
6. Return this crisper plate to the Zone 1 of the Ninja Foodi Dual Zone Air Fryer.
7. Choose the Air Fry mode for Zone 1 and set the temperature to 390 degrees F and the time to 15 minutes.
8. Add potatoes and green beans to the Zone 2.
9. Choose the Air Fry mode for Zone 2 with 350 degrees F and the time to 10 minutes.
10. Press the SYNC button to sync the finish time for both Zones.
11. Initiate cooking by pressing the START/STOP button.
12. Serve the tenderloin with Air Fried potatoes

Nutrition Info:
- (Per serving) Calories 400 | Fat 32g |Sodium 721mg | Carbs 2.6g | Fiber 0g | Sugar 0g | Protein 27.4g

Meatballs

Servings: 4
Cooking Time: 20 Minutes
Ingredients:
- 450g ground beef
- 59ml milk
- 45g parmesan cheese, grated
- 50g breadcrumbs
- ½ tsp Italian seasoning
- 2 garlic cloves, minced
- Pepper
- Salt

Directions:
1. In a bowl, mix the meat and remaining ingredients until well combined.
2. Insert a crisper plate in the Ninja Foodi air fryer baskets.
3. Make small balls from the meat mixture and place them in both baskets.
4. Select zone 1, then select "air fry" mode and set the temperature to 375 degrees F for 15 minutes. Press "match" and "start/stop" to begin.

Nutrition Info:
- (Per serving) Calories 426 | Fat 17.3g |Sodium 820mg | Carbs 11.1g | Fiber 0.7g | Sugar 1.6g | Protein 48.8g

Bell Peppers With Sausages

Servings:4
Cooking Time:20
Ingredients:
- 6 beef or pork Italian sausages
- 4 bell peppers, whole
- Oil spray, for greasing
- 2 cups of cooked rice
- 1 cup of sour cream

Directions:
1. Put the bell pepper in the zone 1 basket and sausages in the zone 2 basket of the air fryer.
2. Set zone 1 to AIR FRY MODE for 10 minutes at 400 degrees F.
3. For zone 2 set it to 20 minutes at 375 degrees F.
4. Hit the smart finish button, so both finish at the same time.
5. After 5 minutes take out the sausage basket and break or mince it with a plastic spatula.
6. Then, let the cooking cycle finish.
7. Once done serve the minced meat with bell peppers and serve over cooked rice with a dollop of sour cream.

Nutrition Info:

- (Per serving) Calories1356 | Fat 81.2g| Sodium 3044 mg | Carbs 96g | Fiber 3.1g | Sugar 8.3g | Protein 57.2 g

Italian-style Meatballs With Garlicky Roasted Broccoli

Servings:4
Cooking Time: 15 Minutes
Ingredients:
- FOR THE MEATBALLS
- 1 large egg
- ¼ cup Italian-style bread crumbs
- 1 pound ground beef (85 percent lean)
- ¼ cup grated Parmesan cheese
- ¼ teaspoon kosher salt
- Nonstick cooking spray
- 2 cups marinara sauce
- FOR THE ROASTED BROCCOLI
- 4 cups broccoli florets
- 1 tablespoon olive oil
- ¼ teaspoon kosher salt
- ¼ teaspoon freshly ground pepper
- ¼ teaspoon red pepper flakes
- 1 tablespoon minced garlic

Directions:
1. To prep the meatballs: In a large bowl, beat the egg. Mix in the bread crumbs and let sit for 5 minutes.
2. Add the beef, Parmesan, and salt and mix until just combined. Form the meatball mixture into 8 meatballs, about 1 inch in diameter. Mist with cooking spray.
3. To prep the broccoli: In a large bowl, combine the broccoli, olive oil, salt, black pepper, and red pepper flakes. Toss to coat the broccoli evenly.
4. To cook the meatballs and broccoli: Install a crisper plate in the Zone 1 basket. Place the meatballs in the basket and insert the basket in the unit. Place the broccoli in the Zone 2 basket, sprinkle the garlic over the broccoli, and insert the basket in the unit.
5. Select Zone 1, select AIR FRY, set the temperature to 400°F, and set the time to 12 minutes.
6. Select Zone 2, select ROAST, set the temperature to 390°F, and set the time to 15 minutes. Select SMART FINISH.
7. Press START/PAUSE to begin cooking.
8. When the Zone 1 timer reads 5 minutes, press START/PAUSE. Remove the basket and pour the marinara sauce over the meatballs. Reinsert the basket and press START/PAUSE to resume cooking.
9. When cooking is complete, the meatballs should be cooked through and the broccoli will have begun to brown on the edges.

Nutrition Info:
- (Per serving) Calories: 493; Total fat: 33g; Saturated fat: 9g; Carbohydrates: 24g; Fiber: 3g; Protein: 31g; Sodium: 926mg

Bacon Wrapped Pork Tenderloin

Servings: 2
Cooking Time: 20 Minutes
Ingredients:
- ½ teaspoon salt
- ¼ teaspoon black pepper
- 1 pork tenderloin
- 6 center cut strips bacon
- cooking string

Directions:
1. Cut two bacon strips in half and place them on the working surface.
2. Place the other bacon strips on top and lay the tenderloin over the bacon strip.
3. Wrap the bacon around the tenderloin and tie the roast with a kitchen string.
4. Place the roast in the first air fryer basket.
5. Return the air fryer basket 1 to Zone 1, and basket 2 to Zone 2 of the Ninja Foodi 2-Basket Air Fryer.
6. Choose the "Air Fry" mode for Zone 1 and set the temperature to 400 degrees F and 20 minutes of cooking time.
7. Initiate cooking by pressing the START/PAUSE BUTTON.
8. Slice and serve warm.

Nutrition Info:
- (Per serving) Calories 459 | Fat 17.7g |Sodium 1516mg | Carbs 1.7g | Fiber 0.5g | Sugar 0.4g | Protein 69.2g

Balsamic Steak Tips With Roasted Asparagus And Mushroom Medley

Servings:4
Cooking Time: 25 Minutes
Ingredients:
- FOR THE STEAK TIPS
- 1½ pounds sirloin tips
- ½ cup olive oil
- ¼ cup balsamic vinegar
- ¼ cup packed light brown sugar
- 1 tablespoon reduced-sodium soy sauce
- 1 teaspoon finely chopped fresh rosemary
- 1 teaspoon minced garlic
- FOR THE ASPARAGUS AND MUSHROOMS
- 6 ounces sliced cremini mushrooms
- 1 small red onion, sliced
- 1 tablespoon olive oil
- 1 pound asparagus, tough ends trimmed
- ⅛ teaspoon kosher salt

Directions:
1. To prep the steak tips: In a large bowl, combine the sirloin tips, oil, vinegar, brown sugar, soy sauce, rosemary, and garlic. Mix well to coat the steak.

2. To prep the mushrooms: In a large bowl, combine the mushrooms, onion, and oil.

3. To cook the steak and vegetables: Install a crisper plate in each of the two baskets. Shake any excess marinade from the steak tips, place the steak in the Zone 1 basket, and insert the basket in the unit. Place the mushrooms and onions in the Zone 2 basket and insert the basket in the unit.

4. Select Zone 1, select AIR FRY, set the temperature to 400°F, and set the time to 12 minutes.

5. Select Zone 2, select ROAST, set the temperature to 400°F, and set the time to 25 minutes. Select SMART FINISH.

6. Press START/PAUSE to begin cooking.

7. When the Zone 2 timer reads 10 minutes, press START/PAUSE. Remove the basket, add the asparagus to the mushrooms and onion, and sprinkle with salt. Reinsert the basket and press START/PAUSE to resume cooking.

8. When cooking is complete, the beef should be cooked to your liking and the asparagus crisp-tender. Serve warm.

Nutrition Info:
- (Per serving) Calories: 524; Total fat: 33g; Saturated fat: 2.5g; Carbohydrates: 16g; Fiber: 3g; Protein: 41g; Sodium: 192mg

Beef Cheeseburgers

Servings: 4
Cooking Time: 13 Minutes.
Ingredients:
- 1 lb. ground beef
- Salt, to taste
- 2 garlic cloves, minced
- 1 tablespoon soy sauce
- Black pepper, to taste
- 4 American cheese slices
- 4 hamburger buns
- Mayonnaise, to serve
- Lettuce, to serve
- Sliced tomatoes, to serve
- Sliced red onion, to serve

Directions:
1. Mix beef with soy sauce and garlic in a large bowl.
2. Make 4 patties of 4 inches in diameter.
3. Rub them with salt and black pepper on both sides.
4. Place the 2 patties in each of the crisper plate.
5. Return the crisper plate to the Ninja Foodi Dual Zone Air Fryer.
6. Choose the Air Fry mode for Zone 1 and set the temperature to 390 degrees F and the time to 13 minutes.
7. Select the "MATCH" button to copy the settings for Zone 2.
8. Initiate cooking by pressing the START/STOP button.
9. Flip each patty once cooked halfway through, and resume cooking.
10. Add each patty to the hamburger buns along with mayo, tomatoes, onions, and lettuce.
11. Serve.

Nutrition Info:
- (Per serving) Calories 437 | Fat 28g |Sodium 1221mg | Carbs 22.3g | Fiber 0.9g | Sugar 8g | Protein 30.3g

Tender Pork Chops

Servings: 2
Cooking Time: 20 Minutes
Ingredients:
- 2 pork chops
- 1 tsp dry mustard
- 1 tsp ground coriander
- 1 tbsp chilli powder
- 30ml olive oil
- ¼ tsp cayenne
- ½ tsp ground cumin
- 1 tsp smoked paprika
- Pepper
- Salt

Directions:
1. In a small bowl, mix chilli powder, paprika, cayenne, coriander, mustard, pepper, and salt.
2. Brush the pork chops with oil and rub with spice mixture.
3. Insert a crisper plate in the Ninja Foodi air fryer baskets.
4. Place the chops in both baskets.
5. Select zone 1, then select "air fry" mode and set the temperature to 375 degrees F for 10 minutes. Press "match" to match zone 2 settings to zone 1. Press "start/stop" to begin. Turn halfway through.

Nutrition Info:
- (Per serving) Calories 401 | Fat 35.3g |Sodium 173mg | Carbs 3.6g | Fiber 2g | Sugar 0.5g | Protein 19.1g

Pork Chops With Brussels Sprouts

Servings: 4
Cooking Time: 15 Minutes.
Ingredients:
- 4 bone-in center-cut pork chop
- Cooking spray
- Salt, to taste
- Black pepper, to taste
- 2 teaspoons olive oil
- 2 teaspoons pure maple syrup
- 2 teaspoons Dijon mustard
- 6 ounces Brussels sprouts, quartered

Directions:
1. Rub pork chop with salt, ¼ teaspoons black pepper, and cooking spray.

2. Toss Brussels sprouts with mustard, syrup, oil, ¼ teaspoon of black pepper in a medium bowl.
3. Add pork chop to the crisper plate of Zone 1 of the Ninja Foodi Dual Zone Air Fryer.
4. Return the crisper plate to the Ninja Foodi Dual Zone Air Fryer.
5. Choose the Air Fry mode for Zone 1 and set the temperature to 400 degrees F and the time to 15 minutes.
6. Add the Brussels sprouts to the crisper plate of Zone 2 and return it to the unit.
7. Choose the Air Fry mode for Zone 2 with 350 degrees F and the time to 13 minutes.
8. Press the SYNC button to sync the finish time for both Zones.
9. Initiate cooking by pressing the START/STOP button.
10. Serve warm and fresh

Nutrition Info:
- (Per serving) Calories 336 | Fat 27.1g |Sodium 66mg | Carbs 1.1g | Fiber 0.4g | Sugar 0.2g | Protein 19.7g

Cinnamon-apple Pork Chops

Servings: 4
Cooking Time: 10 Minutes
Ingredients:
- 2 tablespoons butter
- 4 boneless pork loin chops
- 3 tablespoons brown sugar
- 1 teaspoon ground cinnamon
- ½ teaspoon ground nutmeg
- ¼ teaspoon salt
- 4 medium tart apples, sliced
- 2 tablespoons chopped pecans

Directions:
1. Mix butter, brown sugar, cinnamon, nutmeg, and salt in a bowl.
2. Rub this mixture over the pork chops and place them in the air fryer baskets.
3. Top them with apples and pecans.
4. Return the air fryer basket 1 to Zone 1, and basket 2 to Zone 2 of the Ninja Foodi 2-Basket Air Fryer.
5. Choose the "Air Fry" mode for Zone 1 at 375 degrees F and 10 minutes of cooking time.
6. Select the "MATCH COOK" option to copy the settings for Zone 2.
7. Initiate cooking by pressing the START/PAUSE BUTTON.
8. Serve warm.

Nutrition Info:
- (Per serving) Calories 316 | Fat 17g |Sodium 271mg | Carbs 4.3g | Fiber 0.9g | Sugar 2.1g | Protein 35g

Lamb Shank With Mushroom Sauce

Servings: 4
Cooking Time: 35 Minutes.
Ingredients:
- 20 mushrooms, chopped
- 2 red bell pepper, chopped
- 2 red onion, chopped
- 1 cup red wine
- 4 leeks, chopped
- 6 tablespoons balsamic vinegar
- 2 teaspoons black pepper
- 2 teaspoons salt
- 3 tablespoons fresh rosemary
- 6 garlic cloves
- 4 lamb shanks
- 3 tablespoons olive oil

Directions:
1. Season the lamb shanks with salt, pepper, rosemary, and 1 teaspoon of olive oil.
2. Set half of the shanks in each of the crisper plate.
3. Return the crisper plate to the Ninja Foodi Dual Zone Air Fryer.
4. Choose the Air Fry mode for Zone 1 and set the temperature to 390 degrees F and the time to 25 minutes.
5. Select the "MATCH" button to copy the settings for Zone 2.
6. Initiate cooking by pressing the START/STOP button.
7. Flip the shanks halfway through, and resume cooking.
8. Meanwhile, add and heat the remaining olive oil in a skillet.
9. Add onion and garlic to sauté for 5 minutes.
10. Add in mushrooms and cook for 5 minutes.
11. Add red wine and cook until it is absorbed
12. Stir all the remaining vegetables along with black pepper and salt.
13. Cook until vegetables are al dente.
14. Serve the air fried shanks with sautéed vegetable fry.

Nutrition Info:
- (Per serving) Calories 352 | Fat 9.1g |Sodium 1294mg | Carbs 3.9g | Fiber 1g | Sugar 1g | Protein 61g

Juicy Pork Chops

Servings: 4
Cooking Time: 15 Minutes
Ingredients:
- 450g pork chops
- ¼ tsp garlic powder
- 15ml olive oil
- ¼ tsp smoked paprika
- Pepper
- Salt

Directions:

1. In a small bowl, mix the garlic powder, paprika, pepper, and salt.
2. Brush the pork chops with oil and rub with spice mixture.
3. Insert a crisper plate in the Ninja Foodi air fryer baskets.
4. Place the pork chops in both baskets.
5. Select zone 1, then select "bake" mode and set the temperature to 410 degrees F for 15 minutes. Press "match" to match zone 2 settings to zone 1. Press "start/stop" to begin. Turn halfway through.

Nutrition Info:
- (Per serving) Calories 394 | Fat 31.7g |Sodium 118mg | Carbs 0.2g | Fiber 0.1g | Sugar 0.1g | Protein 25.5g

Chinese Bbq Pork

Servings:35
Cooking Time:25

Ingredients:
- 4 tablespoons of soy sauce
- ¼ cup red wine
- 2 tablespoons of oyster sauce
- ¼ tablespoons of hoisin sauce
- ¼ cup honey
- ¼ cup brown sugar
- Pinch of salt
- Pinch of black pepper
- 1 teaspoon of ginger garlic, paste
- 1 teaspoon of five-spice powder
- 1.5 pounds of pork shoulder, sliced

Directions:
1. Take a bowl and mix all the ingredients listed under sauce ingredients.
2. Transfer half of it to a sauce pan and let it cook for 10 minutes.
3. Set it aside.
4. Let the pork marinate in the remaining sauce for 2 hours.
5. Afterward, put the pork slices in the basket and set it to AIRBORIL mode 450 degrees for 25 minutes.
6. Make sure the internal temperature is above 160 degrees F once cooked.
7. If not add a few more minutes to the overall cooking time.
8. Once done, take it out and baste it with prepared sauce.
9. Serve and Enjoy.

Nutrition Info:
- (Per serving) Calories 1239| Fat 73 g| Sodium 2185 mg | Carbs 57.3 g | Fiber 0.4g| Sugar53.7 g | Protein 81.5 g

Pork Chops With Apples

Servings: 2
Cooking Time: 15 Minutes

Ingredients:
- ½ small red cabbage, sliced
- 1 apple, sliced
- 1 sweet onion, sliced
- 2 tablespoons oil
- ½ teaspoon cumin
- ½ teaspoon paprika
- Salt and black pepper, to taste
- 2 boneless pork chops (1″ thick)

Directions:
1. Toss pork chops with apple and the rest of the ingredients in a bowl.
2. Divide the mixture in the air fryer baskets.
3. Return the air fryer basket 1 to Zone 1, and basket 2 to Zone 2 of the Ninja Foodi 2-Basket Air Fryer.
4. Choose the "Air Fry" mode for Zone 1 and set the temperature to 400 degrees F and 15 minutes of cooking time.
5. Select the "MATCH COOK" option to copy the settings for Zone 2.
6. Initiate cooking by pressing the START/PAUSE BUTTON.
7. Serve warm.

Nutrition Info:
- (Per serving) Calories 374 | Fat 25g |Sodium 275mg | Carbs 7.3g | Fiber 0g | Sugar 6g | Protein 12.3g

Garlic-rosemary Pork Loin With Scalloped Potatoes And Cauliflower

Servings:6
Cooking Time: 50 Minutes

Ingredients:
- FOR THE PORK LOIN
- 2 pounds pork loin roast
- 2 tablespoons vegetable oil
- 2 teaspoons dried thyme
- 2 teaspoons dried crushed rosemary
- 1 teaspoon minced garlic
- ¾ teaspoon kosher salt
- FOR THE SCALLOPED POTATOES AND CAULIFLOWER
- 1 teaspoon vegetable oil
- ¾ pound Yukon Gold potatoes, peeled and very thinly sliced
- 1½ cups cauliflower florets
- ¼ teaspoon kosher salt
- ¼ teaspoon freshly ground black pepper
- 1 tablespoon very cold unsalted butter, grated
- 3 tablespoons all-purpose flour
- 1 cup whole milk
- 1 cup shredded Gruyère cheese

Directions:

1. To prep the pork loin: Coat the pork with the oil. Season with thyme, rosemary, garlic, and salt.
2. To prep the potatoes and cauliflower: Brush the bottom and sides of the Zone 2 basket with the oil. Add one-third of the potatoes to the bottom of the basket and arrange in a single layer. Top with ½ cup of cauliflower florets. Sprinkle a third of the salt and black pepper on top. Scatter one-third of the butter on top and sprinkle on 1 tablespoon of flour. Repeat this step twice more for a total of three layers.
3. Pour the milk over the layered potatoes and cauliflower; it should just cover the top layer. Top with the Gruyère.
4. To cook the pork and scalloped vegetables: Install a crisper plate in the Zone 1 basket. Place the pork loin in the basket and insert the basket in the unit. Insert the Zone 2 basket in the unit.
5. Select Zone 1, select AIR FRY, set the temperature to 390°F, and set the time to 50 minutes.
6. Select Zone 2, select BAKE, set the temperature to 350°F, and set the time to 45 minutes. Select SMART FINISH.
7. Press START/PAUSE to begin cooking.
8. When cooking is complete, the pork will be cooked through (an instant-read thermometer should read 145°F) and the potatoes and cauliflower will be tender.
9. Let the pork rest for at least 15 minutes before slicing and serving with the scalloped vegetables.

Nutrition Info:
- (Per serving) Calories: 439; Total fat: 25g; Saturated fat: 10g; Carbohydrates: 17g; Fiber: 1.5g; Protein: 37g; Sodium: 431mg

Korean Bbq Beef

Servings: 6
Cooking Time: 30 Minutes
Ingredients:
- For the meat:
- 1 pound flank steak or thinly sliced steak
- ¼ cup corn starch
- Coconut oil spray
- For the sauce:
- ½ cup soy sauce or gluten-free soy sauce
- ½ cup brown sugar
- 2 tablespoons white wine vinegar
- 1 clove garlic, crushed
- 1 tablespoon hot chili sauce
- 1 teaspoon ground ginger
- ½ teaspoon sesame seeds
- 1 tablespoon corn starch
- 1 tablespoon water

Directions:
1. To begin, prepare the steak. Thinly slice it in that toss it in the corn starch to be coated thoroughly. Spray the tops with some coconut oil.
2. Spray the crisping plates and drawers with the coconut oil.
3. Place the crisping plates into the drawers. Place the steak strips into each drawer. Insert both drawers into the unit.
4. Select zone 1, Select AIR FRY, set the temperature to 375 degrees F/ 190 degrees C, and set time to 30 minutes. Select MATCH to match zone 2 settings with zone 1. Press the START/STOP button to begin cooking.
5. While the steak is cooking, add the sauce ingredients EXCEPT for the corn starch and water to a medium saucepan.
6. Warm it up to a low boil, then whisk in the corn starch and water.
7. Carefully remove the steak and pour the sauce over. Mix well.

Nutrition Info:
- (Per serving) Calories 500 | Fat 19.8g | Sodium 680mg | Carbs 50.1g | Fiber 4.1g | Sugar 0g | Protein 27.9g

Tasty Pork Skewers

Servings: 3
Cooking Time: 10 Minutes
Ingredients:
- 450g pork shoulder, cut into ¼-inch pieces
- 66ml soy sauce
- ½ tbsp garlic, crushed
- 1 tbsp ginger paste
- 1 ½ tsp sesame oil
- 22ml rice vinegar
- 21ml honey
- Pepper
- Salt

Directions:
1. In a bowl, mix meat with the remaining ingredients. Cover and place in the refrigerator for 30 minutes.
2. Thread the marinated meat onto the soaked skewers.
3. Insert a crisper plate in the Ninja Foodi air fryer baskets.
4. Place the pork skewers in both baskets.
5. Select zone 1, then select "air fry" mode and set the temperature to 360 degrees F for 10 minutes. Press "match" and then press "start/stop" to begin. Turn halfway through.

Nutrition Info:
- (Per serving) Calories 520 | Fat 34.7g |Sodium 1507mg | Carbs 12.2g | Fiber 0.5g | Sugar 9.1g | Protein 37g

Glazed Steak Recipe

Servings: 2
Cooking Time: 25
Ingredients:
- 1 pound of beef steaks
- ½ cup, soy sauce
- Salt and black pepper, to taste
- 1 tablespoon of vegetable oil
- 1 teaspoon of grated ginger
- 4 cloves garlic, minced
- 1/4 cup brown sugar

Directions:
1. Take a bowl and whisk together soy sauce, salt, pepper, vegetable oil, garlic, brown sugar, and ginger.
2. Once a paste is made rub the steak with the marinate
3. Let it sit for 30 minutes.
4. After 30 minutes add the steak to the air fryer basket and set it to AIR BROIL mode at 400 degrees F for 18-22 minutes.
5. After 10 minutes, hit pause and takeout the basket.
6. Let the steak flip and again let it AIR BROIL for the remaining minutes.
7. Once 25 minutes of cooking cycle completes.
8. Take out the steak and let it rest. Serve by cutting into slices.
9. Enjoy.

Nutrition Info:
- (Per serving) Calories 563| Fat 21 g| Sodium 156mg | Carbs 20.6g | Fiber0.3 g| Sugar17.8 g | Protein69.4 g

Pork Chops And Potatoes

Servings: 3
Cooking Time: 12 Minutes
Ingredients:
- 455g red potatoes
- Olive oil
- Salt and pepper
- 1 teaspoon garlic powder
- 1 teaspoon fresh rosemary, chopped
- 2 tablespoons brown sugar
- 1 tablespoon soy sauce
- 1 tablespoon Worcestershire sauce
- 1 teaspoon lemon juice
- 3 small pork chops

Directions:
1. Mix potatoes and pork chops with remaining ingredients in a bowl.
2. Divide the ingredients in the air fryer baskets.
3. Return the air fryer basket 1 to Zone 1, and basket 2 to Zone 2 of the Ninja Foodi 2-Basket Air Fryer.
4. Choose the "Air Fry" mode for Zone 1 at 400 degrees F and 12 minutes of cooking time.
5. Select the "MATCH COOK" option to copy the settings for Zone 2.
6. Initiate cooking by pressing the START/PAUSE BUTTON.
7. Flip the chops and toss potatoes once cooked halfway through.
8. Serve warm.

Nutrition Info:
- (Per serving) Calories 352 | Fat 9.1g |Sodium 1294mg | Carbs 3.9g | Fiber 1g | Sugar 1g | Protein 61g

Beef Ribs I

Servings: 2
Cooking Time: 15
Ingredients:
- 4 tablespoons of barbecue spice rub
- 1 tablespoon kosher salt and black pepper
- 3 tablespoons brown sugar
- 2 pounds of beef ribs (3-3 1/2 pounds), cut in thirds
- 1 cup barbecue sauce

Directions:
1. In a small bowl, add salt, pepper, brown sugar, and BBQ spice rub.
2. Grease the ribs with oil spray from both sides and then rub it with a spice mixture.
3. Divide the ribs amongst the basket and set it to AIR FRY MODE at 375 degrees F for 15 minutes.
4. Hit start and let the air fryer cook the ribs.
5. Once done, serve with the coating BBQ sauce.

Nutrition Info:
- (Per serving) Calories1081 | Fat 28.6 g| Sodium 1701mg | Carbs 58g | Fiber 0.8g| Sugar 45.7g | Protein 138 g

Paprika Pork Chops

Servings: 4
Cooking Time: 12 Minutes
Ingredients:
- 4 bone-in pork chops (6–8 ounces each)
- 1½ tablespoons brown sugar
- 1¼ teaspoons kosher salt
- 1 teaspoon dried Italian seasoning
- 1 teaspoon smoked paprika
- ¼ teaspoon garlic powder
- ¼ teaspoon onion powder
- ¼ teaspoon black pepper
- 1 teaspoon sweet paprika
- 3 tablespoons butter, melted
- 2 tablespoons chopped fresh parsley
- Cooking spray

Directions:
1. In a small mixing bowl, combine the brown sugar, salt, Italian seasoning, smoked paprika, garlic powder, onion powder, black pepper, and sweet paprika. Mix thoroughly.
2. Brush the pork chops on both sides with the melted butter.

3. Rub the spice mixture all over the meat on both sides.
4. Install a crisper plate in both drawers. Place half the chops in the zone 1 drawer and half in zone 2's, then insert the drawers into the unit.
5. Select zone 1, select AIR FRY, set temperature to 390 degrees F/ 200 degrees C, and set time to 12 minutes. Select MATCH to match zone 2 settings to zone 1. Press the START/STOP button to begin cooking.
6. When the time reaches 10 minutes, press START/STOP to pause the unit. Remove the drawers and flip the chops. Re-insert the drawers into the unit and press START/STOP to resume cooking.
7. Serve and enjoy!

Nutrition Info:
- (Per serving) Calories 338 | Fat 21.2g | Sodium 1503mg | Carbs 5.1g | Fiber 0.3g | Sugar 4.6g | Protein 29.3g

Sausage Meatballs

Servings: 24
Cooking Time: 10 Minutes
Ingredients:
- 1 egg, lightly beaten
- 900g pork sausage
- 29g breadcrumbs
- 100g pimientos, drained & diced
- 1 tsp curry powder
- 1 tbsp garlic, minced
- 30ml olive oil
- 1 tbsp fresh rosemary, minced
- 25g parsley, minced
- Pepper
- Salt

Directions:
1. In a bowl, add pork sausage and remaining ingredients and mix until well combined.
2. Insert a crisper plate in the Ninja Foodi air fryer baskets.
3. Make small balls from the meat mixture and place them in both baskets.
4. Select zone 1 then select "air fry" mode and set the temperature to 390 degrees F for 10 minutes. Press "match" to match zone 2 settings to zone 1. Press "start/stop" to begin.

Nutrition Info:
- (Per serving) Calories 153 | Fat 12.2g |Sodium 303mg | Carbs 2.6g | Fiber 0.4g | Sugar 1.1g | Protein 8g

Breaded Pork Chops

Servings: 4
Cooking Time: 10 Minutes
Ingredients:
- 4 boneless, center-cut pork chops, 1-inch thick
- 1 teaspoon Cajun seasoning
- 1½ cups cheese and garlic-flavored croutons
- 2 eggs
- Cooking spray

Directions:
1. Season both sides of the pork chops with the Cajun seasoning on a platter.
2. In a small food processor, pulse the croutons until finely chopped; transfer to a shallow plate.
3. In a separate shallow bowl, lightly beat the eggs.
4. Dip the pork chops in the egg, allowing any excess to drip off. Then place the chops in the crouton crumbs. Coat the chops in cooking spray.
5. Install a crisper plate in both drawers. Place half the pork chops in the zone 1 drawer and half in zone 2's, then insert the drawers into the unit.
6. Select zone 1, select ROAST, set temperature to 390 degrees F/ 200 degrees C, and set time to 10 minutes. Select MATCH to match zone 2 settings to zone 1. Press the START/STOP button to begin cooking.
7. When the time reaches 6 minutes, press START/STOP to pause the unit. Remove the drawers and flip the chops. Reinsert the drawers into the unit and press START/STOP to resume cooking.
8. When cooking is complete, serve and enjoy!

Nutrition Info:
- (Per serving) Calories 394 | Fat 18.1g | Sodium 428mg | Carbs 10g | Fiber 0.8g | Sugar 0.9g | Protein 44.7g

Roast Beef

Servings: 4
Cooking Time: 35 Minutes
Ingredients:
- 2 pounds beef roast
- 1 tablespoon olive oil
- 1 medium onion (optional)
- 1 teaspoon salt
- 2 teaspoons rosemary and thyme, chopped (fresh or dried)

Directions:
1. Combine the sea salt, rosemary, and oil in a large, shallow dish.
2. Using paper towels, pat the meat dry. Place it on a dish and turn it to coat the outside with the oil-herb mixture.
3. Peel the onion and split it in half (if using).
4. Install a crisper plate in both drawers. Place half the beef roast and half an onion in the zone 1 drawer and half the beef and half the onion in zone 2's, then insert the drawers into the unit.
5. Select zone 1, select AIR FRY, set temperature to 360 degrees F/ 180 degrees C, and set time to 22 minutes. Select MATCH to match zone 2 settings to zone 1. Press the START/STOP button to begin cooking.
6. When the time reaches 11 minutes, press START/STOP to pause the unit. Remove the drawers and flip the roast. Re-insert the drawers into the unit and press START/STOP to resume cooking.

Nutrition Info:
- (Per serving) Calories 463 | Fat 17.8g | Sodium 732mg | Carbs 2.8g | Fiber 0.7g | Sugar 1.2g | Protein 69g

Chipotle Beef

Servings: 4
Cooking Time: 18 Minutes.
Ingredients:
- 1 lb. beef steak, cut into chunks
- 1 large egg
- ½ cup parmesan cheese, grated
- ½ cup pork panko
- ½ teaspoon seasoned salt
- Chipotle Ranch Dip
- ¼ cup mayonnaise
- ¼ cup sour cream
- 1 teaspoon chipotle paste
- ½ teaspoon ranch dressing mix
- ¼ medium lime, juiced

Directions:
1. Mix all the ingredients for chipotle ranch dip in a bowl.
2. Keep it in the refrigerator for 30 minutes.
3. Mix pork panko with salt and parmesan.
4. Beat egg in one bowl and spread the panko mixture in another flat bowl.
5. Dip the steak chunks in the egg first, then coat them with panko mixture.
6. Spread them in the two crisper plates and spray them with cooking oil.
7. Return the crisper plate to the Ninja Foodi Dual Zone Air Fryer.
8. Choose the Air Fry mode for Zone 1 and set the temperature to 390 degrees F and the time to 18 minutes.
9. Select the "MATCH" button to copy the settings for Zone 2.
10. Initiate cooking by pressing the START/STOP button.
11. Serve with chipotle ranch and salt and pepper on top. Enjoy.

Nutrition Info:
- (Per serving) Calories 310 | Fat 17g |Sodium 271mg | Carbs 4.3g | Fiber 0.9g | Sugar 2.1g | Protein 35g

Steak Bites With Cowboy Butter

Servings: 4
Cooking Time: 15 Minutes
Ingredients:
- 455g steak sirloin
- Cooking spray
- Cowboy butter sauce
- 1 stick salted butter melted
- 1 tablespoon lemon zest
- 1 tablespoon lemon juice
- ½ teaspoon garlic powder
- ¼ teaspoon red pepper flakes
- ½ teaspoon sea salt
- ½ teaspoon black pepper
- ½ tablespoon Dijon mustard
- ½ teaspoon Worcestershire sauce
- 1 tablespoon parsley freshly chopped

Directions:
1. Mix all the cowboy butter ingredients in a bowl.
2. Stir in steak cubes and mix well.
3. Cover and marinate in the refrigerator for 1 hour.
4. Divide the steak cubes in the air fryer baskets then use cooking spray.
5. Return the air fryer basket 1 to Zone 1, and basket 2 to Zone 2 of the Ninja Foodi 2-Basket Air Fryer.
6. Choose the "Air Fry" mode for Zone 1 at 400 degrees F and 15 minutes of cooking time.
7. Select the "MATCH COOK" option to copy the settings for Zone 2.
8. Initiate cooking by pressing the START/PAUSE BUTTON.
9. Serve warm.

Nutrition Info:
- (Per serving) Calories 264 | Fat 17g |Sodium 129mg | Carbs 0.9g | Fiber 0.3g | Sugar 0g | Protein 27g

Poultry Recipes

Buttermilk Fried Chicken

Servings: 6
Cooking Time: 30 Minutes
Ingredients:
- 1½ pounds boneless, skinless chicken thighs
- 2 cups buttermilk
- 1 cup all-purpose flour
- 1 tablespoon seasoned salt
- ½ tablespoon ground black pepper
- 1 cup panko breadcrumbs
- Cooking spray

Directions:
1. Place the chicken thighs in a shallow baking dish. Cover with the buttermilk. Refrigerate for 4 hours or overnight.
2. In a large gallon-sized resealable bag, combine the flour, seasoned salt, and pepper.
3. Remove the chicken from the buttermilk but don't discard the mixture.
4. Add the chicken to the bag and shake well to coat.
5. Dip the thighs in the buttermilk again, then coat in the panko breadcrumbs.
6. Install a crisper plate in each drawer. Place half the chicken thighs in the zone 1 drawer and half in zone 2's, then insert the drawers into the unit.
7. Select zone 1, select AIR FRY, set temperature to 390 degrees F/ 200 degrees C, and set time to 30 minutes. Select MATCH to match zone 2 settings to zone 1. Press the START/STOP button to begin cooking.
8. When the time reaches 15 minutes, press START/STOP to pause the unit. Remove the drawers and flip the chicken. Re-insert the drawers into the unit and press START/STOP to resume cooking.
9. When cooking is complete, remove the chicken.

Nutrition Info:
- (Per serving) Calories 335 | Fat 12.8g | Sodium 687mg | Carbs 33.1g | Fiber 0.4g | Sugar 4g | Protein 24.5g

Ranch Turkey Tenders With Roasted Vegetable Salad

Servings: 4
Cooking Time: 20 Minutes
Ingredients:
- FOR THE TURKEY TENDERS
- 1 pound turkey tenderloin
- ¼ cup ranch dressing
- ½ cup panko bread crumbs
- Nonstick cooking spray
- FOR THE VEGETABLE SALAD
- 1 large sweet potato, peeled and diced
- 1 zucchini, diced
- 1 red bell pepper, diced
- 1 small red onion, sliced
- 1 tablespoon vegetable oil
- ¼ teaspoon kosher salt
- ½ teaspoon freshly ground black pepper
- 2 cups baby spinach
- ½ cup store-bought balsamic vinaigrette
- ¼ cup chopped walnuts

Directions:
1. To prep the turkey tenders: Slice the turkey crosswise into 16 strips. Brush both sides of each strip with ranch dressing, then coat with the panko. Press the bread crumbs into the turkey to help them adhere. Mist both sides of the strips with cooking spray.
2. To prep the vegetables: In a large bowl, combine the sweet potato, zucchini, bell pepper, onion, and vegetable oil. Stir well to coat the vegetables. Season with the salt and black pepper.
3. To cook the turkey and vegetables: Install a crisper plate in the Zone 1 basket. Place the turkey tenders in the basket in a single layer and insert the basket in the unit. Place the vegetables in the Zone 2 basket and insert the basket in the unit.
4. Select Zone 1, select AIR FRY, set the temperature to 375°F, and set the time to 20 minutes.
5. Select Zone 2, select ROAST, set the temperature to 400°F, and set the time to 20 minutes. Select SMART FINISH.
6. Press START/PAUSE to begin cooking.
7. When both timers read 10 minutes, press START/PAUSE. Remove the Zone 1 basket and use silicone-tipped tongs to flip the turkey tenders. Reinsert the basket in the unit. Remove the Zone 2 basket and shake to redistribute the vegetables. Reinsert the basket and press START/PAUSE to resume cooking.
8. When cooking is complete, the turkey will be golden brown and cooked through (an instant-read thermometer should read 165°F) and the vegetables will be fork-tender.
9. Place the spinach in a large serving bowl. Mix in the roasted vegetables and balsamic vinaigrette. Sprinkle with walnuts. Serve warm with the turkey tenders.

Nutrition Info:
- (Per serving) Calories: 470; Total fat: 28g; Saturated fat: 2.5g; Carbohydrates: 28g; Fiber: 4g; Protein: 31g; Sodium: 718mg

Spicy Chicken Sandwiches With "fried" Pickles

Servings: 4
Cooking Time: 18 Minutes
Ingredients:
- FOR THE CHICKEN SANDWICHES
- 2 tablespoons all-purpose flour
- 2 large eggs
- 2 teaspoons Louisiana-style hot sauce
- 1 cup panko bread crumbs
- 1 teaspoon paprika
- ½ teaspoon garlic powder
- ¼ teaspoon salt
- ¼ teaspoon freshly ground black pepper
- ¼ teaspoon cayenne pepper (optional)
- 4 thin-sliced chicken cutlets (4 ounces each)
- 2 teaspoons vegetable oil
- 4 hamburger rolls
- FOR THE PICKLES
- 1 cup dill pickle chips, drained
- 1 large egg
- ½ cup panko bread crumbs
- Nonstick cooking spray
- ½ cup ranch dressing, for serving (optional)

Directions:
1. To prep the sandwiches: Set up a breading station with three small shallow bowls. Place the flour in the first bowl. In the second bowl, whisk together the eggs and hot sauce. Combine the panko, paprika, garlic powder, salt, black pepper, and cayenne pepper (if using) in the third bowl.
2. Bread the chicken cutlets in this order: First, dip them into the flour, coating both sides. Then, dip into the egg mixture. Finally, coat them in the panko mixture, gently pressing the breading into the chicken to help it adhere. Drizzle the cutlets with the oil.
3. To prep the pickles: Pat the pickles dry with a paper towel.
4. In a small shallow bowl, whisk the egg. Add the panko to a second shallow bowl.
5. Dip the pickles in the egg, then the panko. Mist both sides of the pickles with cooking spray.
6. To cook the chicken and pickles: Install a crisper plate in each of the two baskets. Place the chicken in the Zone 1 basket and insert the basket in the unit. Place the pickles in the Zone 2 basket and insert the basket in the unit.
7. Select Zone 1, select AIR FRY, set the temperature to 390°F, and set the time to 18 minutes.
8. Select Zone 2, select AIR FRY, set the temperature to 400°F, and set the time to 15 minutes. Select SMART FINISH.
9. Press START/PAUSE to begin cooking.
10. When both timers read 10 minutes, press START/PAUSE. Remove the Zone 1 basket and use silicone-tipped tongs to flip the chicken. Reinsert the basket. Remove the Zone 2 basket and shake to redistribute the pickles. Reinsert the basket and press START/PAUSE to resume cooking.
11. When cooking is complete, the breading will be crisp and golden brown and the chicken cooked through (an instant-read thermometer should read 165°F). Place one chicken cutlet on each hamburger roll. Serve the "fried" pickles on the side with ranch dressing, if desired.

Nutrition Info:
- (Per serving) Calories: 418; Total fat: 12g; Saturated fat: 1.5g; Carbohydrates: 42g; Fiber: 2g; Protein: 36g; Sodium: 839mg

Chicken Parmesan With Roasted Lemon-parmesan Broccoli

Servings: 4
Cooking Time: 18 Minutes
Ingredients:
- FOR THE CHICKEN PARMESAN
- 2 tablespoons all-purpose flour
- 2 large eggs
- 1 cup panko bread crumbs
- 2 tablespoons grated Parmesan cheese
- 2 teaspoons Italian seasoning
- 4 thin-sliced chicken cutlets (4 ounces each)
- 2 tablespoons vegetable oil
- ½ cup marinara sauce
- ½ cup shredded part-skim mozzarella cheese
- FOR THE BROCCOLI
- 4 cups broccoli florets
- 2 tablespoons olive oil, divided
- ¼ teaspoon kosher salt
- ¼ teaspoon freshly ground black pepper
- 2 teaspoons fresh lemon juice
- 2 tablespoons grated Parmesan cheese

Directions:
1. To prep the chicken Parmesan: Set up a breading station with 3 small shallow bowls. Place the flour in the first bowl. In the second bowl, beat the eggs. Combine the panko, Parmesan, and Italian seasoning in the third bowl.
2. Bread the chicken cutlets in this order: First, dip them into the flour, coating both sides. Then, dip into the beaten egg. Finally, place in the panko mixture, coating both sides of the cutlets. Drizzle the oil over the cutlets.
3. To prep the broccoli: In a large bowl, combine the broccoli, 1 tablespoon of olive oil, the salt, and black pepper.
4. To cook the chicken and broccoli: Install a crisper plate in the Zone 1 basket. Place the chicken in the basket and insert the basket in the unit. Place the

broccoli in the Zone 2 basket and insert the basket in the unit.
5. Select Zone 1, select AIR FRY, set the temperature to 390°F, and set the time to 18 minutes.
6. Select Zone 2, select ROAST, set the temperature to 390°F, and set the time to 15 minutes. Select SMART FINISH.
7. Press START/PAUSE to begin cooking.
8. When the Zone 1 timer reads 10 minutes, press START/PAUSE. Remove the basket and use silicone-tipped tongs to flip the chicken. Reinsert the basket and press START/PAUSE to resume cooking.
9. When the Zone 1 timer reads 2 minutes, press START/PAUSE. Remove the basket and spoon 2 tablespoons of marinara sauce over each chicken cutlet. Sprinkle the mozzarella on top. Reinsert the basket and press START/PAUSE to resume cooking.
10. When cooking is complete, the cheese will be melted and the chicken cooked through (an instant-read thermometer should read 165°F). Transfer the broccoli to a large bowl. Add the lemon juice and Parmesan and toss to coat. Serve the chicken and broccoli warm.

Nutrition Info:
- (Per serving) Calories: 462; Total fat: 22g; Saturated fat: 5g; Carbohydrates: 25g; Fiber: 2.5g; Protein: 37g; Sodium: 838mg

Balsamic Duck Breast

Servings: 2
Cooking Time: 20 Minutes.
Ingredients:
- 2 duck breasts
- 1 teaspoon parsley
- Salt and black pepper, to taste
- Marinade:
- 1 tablespoon olive oil
- ½ teaspoon French mustard
- 1 teaspoon dried garlic
- 2 teaspoons honey
- ½ teaspoon balsamic vinegar

Directions:
1. Mix olive oil, mustard, garlic, honey, and balsamic vinegar in a bowl.
2. Add duck breasts to the marinade and rub well.
3. Place one duck breast in each crisper plate.
4. Return the crisper plates to the Ninja Foodi Dual Zone Air Fryer.
5. Choose the Air Fry mode for Zone 1 and set the temperature to 360 degrees F and the time to 20 minutes.
6. Select the "MATCH" button to copy the settings for Zone 2.
7. Initiate cooking by pressing the START/STOP button.
8. Flip the duck breasts once cooked halfway through, then resume cooking.
9. Serve warm.

Nutrition Info:
- (Per serving) Calories 546 | Fat 33.1g | Sodium 1201mg | Carbs 30g | Fiber 2.4g | Sugar 9.7g | Protein 32g

Wings With Corn On The Cob

Servings: 2
Cooking Time: 40 Minutes
Ingredients:
- 6 chicken wings, skinless
- 2 tablespoons coconut amino
- 2 tablespoons brown sugar
- 1 teaspoon ginger, paste
- ½ inch garlic, minced
- Salt and black pepper to taste
- 2 corn on cobs, small
- Oil spray, for greasing

Directions:
1. Spray the corns with oil spray and season them with salt.
2. Coat the chicken wings with coconut amino, brown sugar, ginger, garlic, salt, and black pepper.
3. Spray the wings with a good amount of oil spray.
4. Put the chicken wings in the zone 1 basket.
5. Put the corn into the zone 2 basket.
6. Select ROAST mode for the chicken wings and set the time to 23 minutes at 400 degrees F/ 200 degrees C.
7. Press 2 and select the AIR FRY mode for the corn and set the time to 40 at 300 degrees F/ 150 degrees C.
8. Once it's done, serve and enjoy.

Nutrition Info:
- (Per serving) Calories 950 | Fat 33.4g | Sodium 592 mg | Carbs 27.4g | Fiber 2.1g | Sugar 11.3 g | Protein 129g

Spicy Chicken Wings

Servings: 8
Cooking Time: 30 Minutes
Ingredients:
- 900g chicken wings
- 1 tsp black pepper
- 12g brown sugar
- 1 tbsp chilli powder
- 57g butter, melted
- 1 tsp smoked paprika
- 1 tsp garlic powder
- 1 tsp salt

Directions:
1. In a bowl, toss chicken wings with remaining ingredients until well coated.
2. Insert a crisper plate in the Ninja Foodi air fryer baskets.
3. Add the chicken wings to both baskets.
4. Select zone 1, then select "air fry" mode and set the temperature to 355 degrees F for 30 minutes. Press

"match" to match zone 2 settings to zone 1. Press "start/stop" to begin. Turn halfway through.
Nutrition Info:
- (Per serving) Calories 276 | Fat 14.4g |Sodium 439mg | Carbs 2.2g | Fiber 0.5g | Sugar 1.3g | Protein 33.1g

Spice-rubbed Chicken Pieces
Servings:6
Cooking Time:40
Ingredients:
- 3 pounds chicken, pieces
- 1 teaspoon sweet paprika
- 1 teaspoon mustard powder
- 1 tablespoon brown sugar, dark
- Salt and black pepper, to taste
- 1 teaspoon Chile powder, New Mexico
- 1 teaspoon oregano, dried
- ¼ teaspoon allspice powder, ground

Directions:
1. Take a bowl and mix dark brown sugar, salt, paprika, mustard powder, oregano, Chile powder, black pepper, and all spice powder.
2. Mix well and rub this spice mixture all over the chicken.
3. Divide the chicken between two air fryer baskets.
4. Oil sprays the meat and then adds it to the air fryer.
5. Now press button1 and button 2 and set the time to 40 minutes at 350 degrees F.
6. Now press start and once the cooking cycle completes, press pause for both the zones.
7. Take out the chicken and serve hot.

Nutrition Info:
- (Per serving) Calories353 | Fat 7.1g| Sodium400 mg | Carbs 2.2g | Fiber0.4 g | Sugar 1.6g | Protein66 g

Glazed Thighs With French Fries
Servings:3
Cooking Time:35
Ingredients:
- 2 tablespoons of Soy Sauce
- Salt, to taste
- 1 teaspoon of Worcestershire Sauce
- 2 teaspoons Brown Sugar
- 1 teaspoon of Ginger, paste
- 1 teaspoon of Garlic, paste
- 6 Boneless Chicken Thighs
- 1 pound of hand-cut potato fries
- 2 tablespoons of canola oil

Directions:
1. Coat the French fries well with canola oil.
2. Season it with salt.
3. In a small bowl, combine the soy sauce, Worcestershire sauce, brown sugar, ginger, and garlic.
4. Place the chicken in this marinade and let it sit for 40 minutes.
5. Put the chicken thighs into the zone 1 basket and fries into the zone 2 basket.
6. Press button 1 for the first basket, and set it to ROAST mode at 350 degrees F for 35 minutes.
7. For the second basket hit 2 and set time to 30 minutes at 360 degrees F, by selecting AIR FRY mode.
8. Once the cooking cycle completely take out the fries and chicken and serve it hot.

Nutrition Info:
- (Per serving) Calories 858| Fat39g | Sodium 1509mg | Carbs 45.6g | Fiber 4.4g | Sugar3 g | Protein 90g

Sweet-and-sour Chicken With Pineapple Cauliflower Rice
Servings:4
Cooking Time: 30 Minutes
Ingredients:
- FOR THE CHICKEN
- ¼ cup cornstarch, plus 2 teaspoons
- ¼ teaspoon kosher salt
- 2 large eggs
- 1 tablespoon sesame oil
- 1½ pounds boneless, skinless chicken breasts, cut into 1-inch pieces
- Nonstick cooking spray
- 6 tablespoons ketchup
- ¾ cup apple cider vinegar
- 1½ tablespoons soy sauce
- 1 tablespoon sugar
- FOR THE CAULIFLOWER RICE
- 1 cup finely diced fresh pineapple
- 1 red bell pepper, thinly sliced
- 1 small red onion, thinly sliced
- 1 tablespoon vegetable oil
- 2 cups frozen cauliflower rice, thawed
- 2 tablespoons soy sauce
- 1 teaspoon sesame oil
- 2 scallions, sliced

Directions:
1. To prep the chicken: Set up a breading station with two small shallow bowls. Combine ¼ cup of cornstarch and the salt in the first bowl. In the second bowl, beat the eggs with the sesame oil.
2. Dip the chicken pieces in the cornstarch mixture to coat, then into the egg mixture, then back into the cornstarch mixture to coat. Mist the coated pieces with cooking spray.
3. In a small bowl, whisk together the ketchup, vinegar, soy sauce, sugar, and remaining 2 teaspoons of cornstarch.
4. To prep the cauliflower rice: Blot the pineapple dry with a paper towel. In a large bowl, combine the pineapple, bell pepper, onion, and vegetable oil.

5. To cook the chicken and cauliflower rice: Install a crisper plate in each of the two baskets. Place the chicken in the Zone 1 basket and insert the basket in the unit. Place a piece of aluminum foil over the crisper plate in the Zone 2 basket and add the pineapple mixture. Insert the basket in the unit.

6. Select Zone 1, select AIR FRY, set the temperature to 400°F, and set the time to 30 minutes.

7. Select Zone 2, select AIR BROIL, set the temperature to 450°F, and set the time to 12 minutes. Select SMART FINISH.

8. Press START/PAUSE to begin cooking.

9. When the Zone 2 timer reads 4 minutes, press START/PAUSE. Remove the basket and stir in the cauliflower rice, soy sauce, and sesame oil. Reinsert the basket and press START/PAUSE to resume cooking.

10. When cooking is complete, the chicken will be golden brown and cooked through and the rice warmed through. Stir the scallions into the rice and serve.

Nutrition Info:
- (Per serving) Calories: 457; Total fat: 17g; Saturated fat: 2.5g; Carbohydrates: 31g; Fiber: 2.5g; Protein: 43g; Sodium: 1,526mg

Asian Chicken

Servings: 4
Cooking Time: 12 Minutes
Ingredients:
- 8 chicken thighs, boneless
- 4 garlic cloves, minced
- 85g honey
- 120ml soy sauce
- 1 tsp dried oregano
- 2 tbsp parsley, chopped
- 1 tbsp ketchup

Directions:
1. Add chicken and remaining ingredients in a bowl and mix until well coated. Cover and place in the refrigerator for 6 hours.
2. Insert a crisper plate in the Ninja Foodi air fryer baskets.
3. Remove the chicken from the marinade and place them in both baskets.
4. Select zone 1 then select "air fry" mode and set the temperature to 390 degrees F for 12 minutes. Press "match" to match zone 2 settings to zone 1. Press "start/stop" to begin.

Nutrition Info:
- (Per serving) Calories 646 | Fat 21.7g |Sodium 2092mg | Carbs 22.2g | Fiber 0.6g | Sugar 18.9g | Protein 86.9g

Sweet And Spicy Carrots With Chicken Thighs

Servings:2
Cooking Time:35
Ingredients:
- Cooking spray, for greasing
- 2 tablespoons butter, melted
- 1 tablespoon hot honey
- 1 teaspoon orange zest
- 1 teaspoon cardamom
- ½ pound baby carrots
- 1 tablespoon orange juice
- Salt and black pepper, to taste
- ½ pound of carrots, baby carrots
- 8 chicken thighs

Directions:
1. Take a bowl and mix all the glaze ingredients in it.
2. Now, coat the chicken and carrots with the glaze and let it rest for 30 minutes.
3. Now place the chicken thighs into the zone 1 basket.
4. Next put the glazed carrots into the zone 2 basket.
5. Press button 1 for the first basket and set it to ROAST Mode at 350 degrees F for 35 minutes.
6. For the second basket hit 2 and set time to AIRFRY mode at 390 degrees F for 8-10 minutes.
7. Once the cooking cycle completes take out the carrots and chicken and serve it hot.

Nutrition Info:
- (Per serving) Calories 1312| Fat 55.4g| Sodium 757mg | Carbs 23.3g | Fiber6.7 g | Sugar12 g | Protein171 g

Marinated Chicken Legs

Servings: 6
Cooking Time: 28 Minutes
Ingredients:
- 6 chicken legs
- 15ml olive oil
- 1 tsp ground mustard
- 36g brown sugar
- ¼ tsp cayenne
- 1 tsp smoked paprika
- 1 tsp garlic powder
- 1 tsp onion powder
- Pepper
- Salt

Directions:
1. Add the chicken legs and the remaining ingredients into a zip-lock bag. Seal the bag and place in the refrigerator for 4 hours.
2. Insert a crisper plate in the Ninja Foodi air fryer baskets.
3. Place the marinated chicken legs in both baskets.
4. Select zone 1, then select "bake" mode and set the temperature to 390 degrees F for 25-28 minutes. Press "match" to match zone 2 settings to zone 1. Press "start/stop" to begin.

Nutrition Info:

- (Per serving) Calories 308 | Fat 17.9g |Sodium 128mg | Carbs 5.5g | Fiber 0.3g | Sugar 4.7g | Protein 29.9g

Thai Curry Chicken Kabobs
Servings: 4
Cooking Time: 15 Minutes
Ingredients:
- 900g skinless chicken thighs
- 120ml Tamari
- 60ml coconut milk
- 3 tablespoons lime juice
- 3 tablespoons maple syrup
- 2 tablespoons Thai red curry

Directions:
1. Mix red curry paste, honey, lime juice, coconut milk, soy sauce in a bowl.
2. Add this sauce and chicken to a Ziplock bag.
3. Seal the bag and shake it to coat well.
4. Refrigerate the chicken for 2 hours then thread the chicken over wooden skewers.
5. Divide the skewers in the air fryer baskets.
6. Return the air fryer basket 1 to Zone 1, and basket 2 to Zone 2 of the Ninja Foodi 2-Basket Air Fryer.
7. Choose the "Air Fry" mode for Zone 1 at 350 degrees F and 15 minutes of cooking time.
8. Select the "MATCH COOK" option to copy the settings for Zone 2.
9. Initiate cooking by pressing the START/PAUSE BUTTON.
10. Flip the skewers once cooked halfway through.
11. Serve warm.

Nutrition Info:
- (Per serving) Calories 353 | Fat 5g |Sodium 818mg | Carbs 53.2g | Fiber 4.4g | Sugar 8g | Protein 17.3g

Bang-bang Chicken
Servings: 2
Cooking Time: 20 Minutes.
Ingredients:
- 1 cup mayonnaise
- ½ cup sweet chili sauce
- 2 tablespoons Sriracha sauce
- ⅓ cup flour
- 1 lb. boneless chicken breast, diced
- 1 ½ cups panko bread crumbs
- 2 green onions, chopped

Directions:
1. Mix mayonnaise with Sriracha and sweet chili sauce in a large bowl.
2. Keep ¾ cup of the mixture aside.
3. Add flour, chicken, breadcrumbs, and remaining mayo mixture to a resealable plastic bag.
4. Zip the bag and shake well to coat.
5. Divide the chicken in the two crisper plates in a single layer.
6. Return the crisper plate to the Ninja Foodi Dual Zone Air Fryer.
7. Choose the Air Fry mode for Zone 1 and set the temperature to 390 degrees F and the time to 20 minutes.
8. Select the "MATCH" button to copy the settings for Zone 2.
9. Initiate cooking by pressing the START/STOP button.
10. Flip the chicken once cooked halfway through.
11. Top the chicken with reserved mayo sauce.
12. Garnish with green onions and serve warm.

Nutrition Info:
- (Per serving) Calories 374 | Fat 13g |Sodium 552mg | Carbs 25g | Fiber 1.2g | Sugar 1.2g | Protein 37.7g

Almond Chicken
Servings: 4
Cooking Time: 25 Minutes
Ingredients:
- 2 large eggs
- ½ cup buttermilk
- 2 teaspoons garlic salt
- 1 teaspoon pepper
- 2 cups slivered almonds, finely chopped
- 4 boneless, skinless chicken breast halves (6 ounces each)

Directions:
1. Whisk together the egg, buttermilk, garlic salt, and pepper in a small bowl.
2. In another small bowl, place the almonds.
3. Dip the chicken in the egg mixture, then roll it in the almonds, patting it down to help the coating stick.
4. Install a crisper plate in both drawers. Place half the chicken breasts in the zone 1 drawer and half in zone 2's, then insert the drawers into the unit.
5. Select zone 1, select AIR FRY, set temperature to 390 degrees F/ 200 degrees C, and set time to 22 minutes. Select MATCH to match zone 2 settings to zone 1. Press the START/STOP button to begin cooking.
6. When the time reaches 11 minutes, press START/STOP to pause the unit. Remove the drawers and flip the chicken. Re-insert the drawers into the unit and press START/STOP to resume cooking.
7. When cooking is complete, remove the chicken.

Nutrition Info:
- (Per serving) Calories 353 | Fat 18g | Sodium 230mg | Carbs 6g | Fiber 2g | Sugar 3g | Protein 41g

Cheddar-stuffed Chicken
Servings: 4
Cooking Time: 20 Minutes.
Ingredients:
- 3 bacon strips, cooked and crumbled
- 2 ounces Cheddar cheese, cubed
- ¼ cup barbeque sauce
- 2 (4 ounces) boneless chicken breasts

- Salt and black pepper to taste

Directions:
1. Make a 1-inch deep pouch in each chicken breast.
2. Mix cheddar cubes with half of the BBQ sauce, salt, black pepper, and bacon.
3. Divide this filling in the chicken breasts and secure the edges with a toothpick.
4. Brush the remaining BBQ sauce over the chicken breasts.
5. Place the chicken in the crisper plate and spray them with cooking oil.
6. Return the crisper plate to the Ninja Foodi Dual Zone Air Fryer.
7. Choose the Air Fry mode for Zone 1 and set the temperature to 360 degrees F and the time to 20 minutes.
8. Initiate cooking by pressing the START/STOP button.
9. Serve warm.

Nutrition Info:
- (Per serving) Calories 379 | Fat 19g |Sodium 184mg | Carbs 12.3g | Fiber 0.6g | Sugar 2g | Protein 37.7g

Goat Cheese–stuffed Chicken Breast With Broiled Zucchini And Cherry Tomatoes

Servings:4
Cooking Time: 25 Minutes

Ingredients:
- FOR THE STUFFED CHICKEN BREASTS
- 2 ounces soft goat cheese
- 1 tablespoon minced fresh parsley
- ½ teaspoon minced garlic
- 4 boneless, skinless chicken breasts (6 ounces each)
- 1 tablespoon vegetable oil
- ½ teaspoon Italian seasoning
- ½ teaspoon kosher salt
- ½ teaspoon freshly ground black pepper
- FOR THE ZUCCHINI AND TOMATOES
- 1 pound zucchini, diced
- 1 cup cherry tomatoes, halved
- 1 tablespoon vegetable oil
- ½ teaspoon kosher salt
- ¼ teaspoon freshly ground black pepper

Directions:
1. To prep the stuffed chicken breasts: In a small bowl, combine the goat cheese, parsley, and garlic. Mix well.
2. Cut a deep slit into the fatter side of each chicken breast to create a pocket (taking care to not go all the way through). Stuff each breast with the goat cheese mixture. Use a toothpick to secure the opening of the chicken, if needed.
3. Brush the outside of the chicken breasts with the oil and season with the Italian seasoning, salt, and black pepper.
4. To prep the zucchini and tomatoes: In a large bowl, combine the zucchini, tomatoes, and oil. Mix to coat. Season with salt and black pepper.
5. To cook the chicken and vegetables: Install a crisper plate in each of the two baskets. Insert a broil rack in the Zone 2 basket over the crisper plate. Place the chicken in the Zone 1 basket and insert the basket in the unit. Place the vegetables on the broiler rack in the Zone 2 basket and insert the basket in the unit.
6. Select Zone 1, select AIR FRY, set the temperature to 390°F, and set the time to 25 minutes.
7. Select Zone 2, select AIR BROIL, set the temperature to 450°F, and set the time to 10 minutes. Select SMART FINISH.
8. Press START/PAUSE to begin cooking.
9. When cooking is complete, the chicken will be golden brown and cooked through (an instant-read thermometer should read 165°F) and the zucchini will be soft and slightly charred. Serve hot.

Nutrition Info:
- (Per serving) Calories: 330; Total fat: 15g; Saturated fat: 4g; Carbohydrates: 5g; Fiber: 1.5g; Protein: 42g; Sodium: 409mg

Air-fried Turkey Breast With Roasted Green Bean Casserole

Servings:4
Cooking Time: 50 Minutes

Ingredients:
- FOR THE TURKEY BREAST
- 2 teaspoons unsalted butter, at room temperature
- 1 bone-in split turkey breast (3 pounds), thawed if frozen
- 1 teaspoon poultry seasoning
- ½ teaspoon kosher salt
- ⅓ teaspoon freshly ground black pepper
- FOR THE GREEN BEAN CASSEROLE
- 1 (10.5-ounce) can condensed cream of mushroom soup
- ½ cup whole milk
- 1 cup store-bought crispy fried onions, divided
- ¼ teaspoon kosher salt
- ¼ teaspoon freshly ground black pepper
- 1 pound green beans, trimmed
- ¼ cup panko bread crumbs
- Nonstick cooking spray

Directions:
1. To prep the turkey breast: Spread the butter over the skin side of the turkey. Season with the poultry seasoning, salt, and black pepper.
2. To prep the green bean casserole: In a medium bowl, combine the soup, milk, ½ cup of crispy onions, the salt, and black pepper.
3. To cook the turkey and beans: Install a crisper plate in the Zone 1 basket. Place the turkey skin-side up in the basket and insert the basket in the unit. Place the green

beans in the Zone 2 basket and insert the basket in the unit.
4. Select Zone 1, select AIR FRY, set the temperature to 360°F, and set the time to 50 minutes.
5. Select Zone 2, select ROAST, set the temperature to 350°F, and set the time to 40 minutes. Select SMART FINISH.
6. Press START/PAUSE to begin cooking.
7. When the Zone 2 timer reads 30 minutes, press START/PAUSE. Remove the basket and stir the soup mixture into the beans. Scatter the panko and remaining ½ cup of crispy onions over the top, then spritz with cooking spray. Reinsert the basket and press START/PAUSE to resume cooking.
8. When cooking is complete, the turkey will be cooked through (an instant-read thermometer should read 165°F) and the green bean casserole will be bubbling and golden brown on top.
9. Let the turkey and casserole rest for at least 15 minutes before serving.
Nutrition Info:
- (Per serving) Calories: 577; Total fat: 22g; Saturated fat: 6.5g; Carbohydrates: 24g; Fiber: 3.5g; Protein: 68g; Sodium: 1,165mg

Chicken Drumettes

Servings: 5
Cooking Time: 52 Minutes.
Ingredients:
- 10 large chicken drumettes
- Cooking spray
- ¼ cup of rice vinegar
- 3 tablespoons honey
- 2 tablespoons unsalted chicken stock
- 1 tablespoon soy sauce
- 1 tablespoon toasted sesame oil
- ⅜ teaspoons crushed red pepper
- 1 garlic clove, chopped
- 2 tablespoons chopped unsalted roasted peanuts
- 1 tablespoon chopped fresh chives

Directions:
1. Spread the chicken in the two crisper plates in an even layer and spray cooking spray on top.
2. Return the crisper plate to the Ninja Foodi Dual Zone Air Fryer.
3. Choose the Air Fry mode for Zone 1 and set the temperature to 390 degrees F and the time to 47 minutes.
4. Select the "MATCH" button to copy the settings for Zone 2.
5. Initiate cooking by pressing the START/STOP button.
6. Flip the chicken drumettes once cooked halfway through, then resume cooking.
7. During this time, mix soy sauce, honey, stock, vinegar, garlic, and crushed red pepper in a suitable saucepan and place it over medium-high heat to cook on a simmer.
8. Cook this sauce for 6 minutes with occasional stirring, then pour it into a medium-sized bowl.
9. Add air fried drumettes and toss well to coat with the honey sauce.
10. Garnish with chives and peanuts.
11. Serve warm and fresh.
Nutrition Info:
- (Per serving) Calories 268 | Fat 10.4g |Sodium 411mg | Carbs 0.4g | Fiber 0.1g | Sugar 0.1g | Protein 40.6g

Chicken Ranch Wraps

Servings: 4
Cooking Time: 22 Minutes
Ingredients:
- 1½ ounces breaded chicken breast tenders
- 4 (12-inch) whole-wheat tortilla wraps
- 2 heads romaine lettuce, chopped
- ½ cup shredded mozzarella cheese
- 4 tablespoons ranch dressing

Directions:
1. Place a crisper plate in each drawer. Place half of the chicken tenders in one drawer and half in the other. Insert the drawers into the unit.
2. Select zone 1, then AIR FRY, and set the temperature to 390 degrees F/ 200 degrees C with a 22-minute timer. To match zone 2 settings to zone 1, choose MATCH. To begin cooking, press the START/STOP button.
3. To pause the unit, press START/STOP when the timer reaches 11 minutes. Remove the drawers from the unit and flip the tenders over. To resume cooking, re-insert the drawers into the device and press START/STOP.
4. Remove the chicken from the drawers when they're done cooking and chop them up.
5. Divide the chopped chicken between warmed-up wraps. Top with some lettuce, cheese, and ranch dressing. Wrap and serve.
Nutrition Info:
- (Per serving) Calories 212 | Fat 7.8g | Sodium 567mg | Carbs 9.1g | Fiber 34.4g | Sugar 9.7g | Protein 10.6g

Easy Chicken Thighs

Servings: 8
Cooking Time: 12 Minutes
Ingredients:
- 900g chicken thighs, boneless & skinless
- 2 tsp chilli powder
- 2 tsp olive oil
- 1 tsp garlic powder
- 1 tsp ground cumin
- Pepper

- Salt

Directions:
1. In a bowl, mix chicken with remaining ingredients until well coated.
2. Insert a crisper plate in the Ninja Foodi air fryer baskets.
3. Place chicken thighs in both baskets.
4. Select zone 1 then select "air fry" mode and set the temperature to 390 degrees F for 12 minutes. Press "match" to match zone 2 settings to zone 1. Press "start/stop" to begin. Turn halfway through.

Nutrition Info:
- (Per serving) Calories 230 | Fat 9.7g |Sodium 124mg | Carbs 0.7g | Fiber 0.3g | Sugar 0.2g | Protein 33g

Greek Chicken Meatballs

Servings: 4
Cooking Time: 9 Minutes
Ingredients:
- 455g ground chicken
- 1 large egg
- 1½ tablespoons garlic paste
- 1 tablespoon dried oregano
- 1 teaspoon lemon zest
- 1 teaspoon dried onion powder
- ¾ teaspoon salt
- ¼ teaspoon black pepper
- Oil spray

Directions:
1. Mix ground chicken with rest of the ingredients in a bowl.
2. Make 1-inch sized meatballs out of this mixture.
3. Place the meatballs in the air fryer baskets.
4. Return the air fryer basket 1 to Zone 1, and basket 2 to Zone 2 of the Ninja Foodi 2-Basket Air Fryer.
5. Choose the "Air Fry" mode for Zone 1 and set the temperature to 390 degrees F and 9 minutes of cooking time.
6. Select the "MATCH COOK" option to copy the settings for Zone 2.
7. Initiate cooking by pressing the START/PAUSE BUTTON.
8. Serve warm.

Nutrition Info:
- (Per serving) Calories 346 | Fat 16.1g |Sodium 882mg | Carbs 1.3g | Fiber 0.5g | Sugar 0.5g | Protein 48.2g

Coconut Chicken Tenders With Broiled Utica Greens

Servings: 4
Cooking Time: 25 Minutes
Ingredients:
- FOR THE CHICKEN TENDERS
- 2 tablespoons all-purpose flour
- 2 large eggs
- 1 cup unsweetened shredded coconut
- ¾ cup panko bread crumbs
- ½ teaspoon kosher salt
- 1½ pounds chicken tenders
- Nonstick cooking spray
- FOR THE UTICA GREENS
- 12 ounces frozen chopped escarole or Swiss chard, thawed and drained
- ¼ cup diced prosciutto
- 2 tablespoons chopped pickled cherry peppers
- ½ teaspoon garlic powder
- ½ teaspoon onion powder
- ¼ teaspoon kosher salt
- ¼ cup Italian-style bread crumbs
- ¼ cup grated Romano cheese
- Nonstick cooking spray

Directions:
1. To prep the chicken tenders: Set up a breading station with three small shallow bowls. Place the flour in the first bowl. In the second bowl, beat the eggs. Combine the coconut, bread crumbs, and salt in the third bowl.
2. Bread the chicken tenders in this order: First, coat them in the flour. Then, dip into the beaten egg. Finally, coat them in the coconut breading, gently pressing the breading into the chicken to help it adhere. Mist both sides of each tender with cooking spray.
3. To prep the Utica greens: In the Zone 2 basket, mix the greens, prosciutto, cherry peppers, garlic powder, onion powder, and salt. Scatter the bread crumbs and Romano cheese over the top. Spritz the greens with cooking spray.
4. To cook the chicken and greens: Install a crisper plate in the Zone 1 basket. Place the chicken tenders in the basket in a single layer and insert the basket in the unit. Insert the Zone 2 basket in the unit.
5. Select Zone 1, select AIR FRY, set the temperature to 390°F, and set the time to 25 minutes.
6. Select Zone 2, select AIR BROIL, set the temperature to 450°F, and set the time to 10 minutes. Select SMART FINISH.
7. Press START/PAUSE to begin cooking.
8. When cooking is complete, the chicken will be crispy and cooked through (an instant-read thermometer should read 165°F) and the greens should be warmed through and toasted on top. Serve warm.

Nutrition Info:
- (Per serving) Calories: 527; Total fat: 26g; Saturated fat: 11g; Carbohydrates: 24g; Fiber: 6.5g; Protein: 50g; Sodium: 886mg

Roasted Garlic Chicken Pizza With Cauliflower "wings"

Servings: 4
Cooking Time: 25 Minutes
Ingredients:
- FOR THE PIZZA
- 2 prebaked rectangular pizza crusts or flatbreads
- 2 tablespoons olive oil
- 1 tablespoon minced garlic
- 1½ cups shredded part-skim mozzarella cheese
- 6 ounces boneless, skinless chicken breast, thinly sliced
- ¼ teaspoon red pepper flakes (optional)
- FOR THE CAULIFLOWER "WINGS"
- 4 cups cauliflower florets
- 1 tablespoon vegetable oil
- ½ cup Buffalo wing sauce

Directions:
1. To prep the pizza: Trim the pizza crusts to fit in the air fryer basket, if necessary.
2. Brush the top of each crust with the oil and sprinkle with the garlic. Top the crusts with the mozzarella, chicken, and red pepper flakes (if using).
3. To prep the cauliflower "wings": In a large bowl, combine the cauliflower and oil and toss to coat the florets.
4. To cook the pizza and "wings": Install a crisper plate in each of the two baskets. Place one pizza in the Zone 1 basket and insert the basket in the unit. Place the cauliflower in the Zone 2 basket and insert the basket in the unit.
5. Select Zone 1, select ROAST, set the temperature to 375°F, and set the time to 25 minutes.
6. Select Zone 2, select AIR FRY, set the temperature to 390°F, and set the time to 25 minutes. Select SMART FINISH.
7. Press START/PAUSE to begin cooking.
8. When the Zone 1 timer reads 13 minutes, press START/PAUSE. Remove the basket. Transfer the pizza to a cutting board (the chicken should be cooked through and the cheese melted and bubbling). Add the second pizza to the basket. Reinsert the basket in the unit and press START/PAUSE to resume cooking.
9. When the Zone 2 timer reads 5 minutes, press START/PAUSE. Remove the basket and add the Buffalo wing sauce to the cauliflower. Shake well to evenly coat the cauliflower in the sauce. Reinsert the basket and press START/PAUSE to resume cooking.
10. When cooking is complete, the cauliflower will be crisp on the outside and tender inside, and the chicken on the second pizza will be cooked through and the cheese melted.
11. Cut each pizza into 4 slices. Serve with the cauliflower "wings" on the side.

Nutrition Info:
- (Per serving) Calories: 360; Total fat: 20g; Saturated fat: 6.5g; Carbohydrates: 21g; Fiber: 2.5g; Protein: 24g; Sodium: 1,399mg

Cajun Chicken With Vegetables

Servings: 6
Cooking Time: 20 Minutes
Ingredients:
- 450g chicken breast, boneless & diced
- 1 tbsp Cajun seasoning
- 400g grape tomatoes
- ⅛ tsp dried thyme
- ⅛ tsp dried oregano
- 1 tsp smoked paprika
- 1 zucchini, diced
- 30ml olive oil
- 1 bell pepper, diced
- 1 tsp onion powder
- 1 ½ tsp garlic powder
- Pepper
- Salt

Directions:
1. In a bowl, toss chicken with vegetables, oil, herb, spices, and salt until well coated.
2. Insert a crisper plate in the Ninja Foodi air fryer baskets.
3. Add chicken and vegetable mixture to both baskets.
4. Select zone 1, then select "air fry" mode and set the temperature to 390 degrees F for 20 minutes. Press "match" to match zone 2 settings to zone 1. Press "start/stop" to begin.

Nutrition Info:
- (Per serving) Calories 153 | Fat 6.9g | Sodium 98mg | Carbs 6g | Fiber 1.6g | Sugar 3.5g | Protein 17.4g

"fried" Chicken With Warm Baked Potato Salad

Servings: 4
Cooking Time: 40 Minutes
Ingredients:
- FOR THE "FRIED" CHICKEN
- 1 cup buttermilk
- 1 tablespoon kosher salt
- 4 bone-in, skin-on chicken drumsticks and/or thighs
- 2 cups all-purpose flour
- 1 tablespoon seasoned salt
- 1 tablespoon paprika
- Nonstick cooking spray
- FOR THE POTATO SALAD
- 1½ pounds baby red potatoes, halved
- 1 tablespoon vegetable oil
- ½ cup mayonnaise
- ⅓ cup plain reduced-fat Greek yogurt
- 1 tablespoon apple cider vinegar

- ½ teaspoon kosher salt
- ½ teaspoon freshly ground black pepper
- ¾ cup shredded Cheddar cheese
- 4 slices cooked bacon, crumbled
- 3 scallions, sliced

Directions:
1. To prep the chicken: In a large bowl, combine the buttermilk and salt. Add the chicken and turn to coat. Let rest for at least 30 minutes (for the best flavor, marinate the chicken overnight in the refrigerator).
2. In a separate large bowl, combine the flour, seasoned salt, and paprika.
3. Remove the chicken from the marinade and allow any excess marinade to drip off. Discard the marinade. Dip the chicken pieces in the flour, coating them thoroughly. Mist with cooking spray. Let the chicken rest for 10 minutes.
4. To prep the potatoes: In a large bowl, combine the potatoes and oil and toss to coat.
5. To cook the chicken and potatoes: Install a crisper plate in the Zone 1 basket. Place the chicken in the basket in a single layer and insert the basket in the unit. Place the potatoes in the Zone 2 basket and insert the basket in the unit.
6. Select Zone 1, select AIR FRY, set the temperature to 390°F, and set the time to 30 minutes.
7. Select Zone 2, select BAKE, set the temperature to 400°F, and set the time to 40 minutes. Select SMART FINISH.
8. Press START/PAUSE to begin cooking.
9. When cooking is complete, the chicken will be golden brown and cooked through (an instant-read thermometer should read 165°F) and the potatoes will be fork-tender.
10. Rinse the potatoes under cold water for about 1 minute to cool them.
11. Place the potatoes in a large bowl and stir in the mayonnaise, yogurt, vinegar, salt, and black pepper. Gently stir in the Cheddar, bacon, and scallions. Serve warm with the "fried" chicken.

Nutrition Info:
- (Per serving) Calories: 639; Total fat: 38g; Saturated fat: 9.5g; Carbohydrates: 54g; Fiber: 4g; Protein: 21g; Sodium: 1,471mg

Cornish Hen With Asparagus

Servings:2
Cooking Time:45
Ingredients:
- 10 spears of asparagus
- Salt and black pepper, to taste
- 1 Cornish hen
- Salt, to taste
- Black pepper, to taste
- 1 teaspoon of Paprika
- Coconut spray, for greasing
- 2 lemons, sliced

Directions:
1. Wash and pat dry the asparagus and coat it with coconut oil spray.
2. Sprinkle salt on the asparagus and place inside the first basket of the air fryer.
3. Next, take the Cornish hen and rub it well with the salt, black pepper, and paprika.
4. Oil sprays the Cornish hen and place in the second air fryer basket.
5. Press button 1 for the first basket and set it to AIR FRY mode at 350 degrees F, for 8 minutes.
6. For the second basket hit 2 and set the time to 45 minutes at 350 degrees F, by selecting the ROAST mode.
7. To start cooking, hit the smart finish button and press hit start.
8. Once the 6 minutes pass press 1 and pause and take out the asparagus.
9. Once the chicken cooking cycle complete, press 2 and hit pause.
10. Take out the Basket of chicken and let it transfer to the serving plate
11. Serve the chicken with roasted asparagus and slices of lemon.
12. Serve hot and enjoy.

Nutrition Info:
- (Per serving) Calories 192| Fat 4.7g| Sodium 151mg | Carbs10.7 g | Fiber 4.6g | Sugar 3.8g | Protein 30g

Chicken Kebabs

Servings: 4
Cooking Time: 9 Minutes
Ingredients:
- 455g boneless chicken breast, cut into 1-inch pieces
- 1 tablespoon avocado oil
- 1 tablespoon Tamari soy sauce
- 1 teaspoon garlic powder
- 1 teaspoon ground ginger
- 1 teaspoon chili powder
- 1 tablespoon honey
- 1 green capsicum, cut into 1-inch pieces
- 1 red capsicum, cut into 1-inch pieces
- 1 yellow capsicum, cut into 1-inch pieces
- 1 courgette, cut into 1-inch pieces
- 1 small red onion, cut into 1-inch pieces
- cooking spray

Directions:
1. Rub chicken with oil and place in a bowl.
2. Mix honey, chili powder, ginger, garlic and soy sauce in a bowl.
3. Pour this mixture over the chicken.
4. Cover and marinate the chicken for 15 minutes.
5. Thread the marinated chicken with veggies on wooden skewers alternately.
6. Divide the skewers and place in the air fryer baskets.

7. Return the air fryer basket 1 to Zone 1, and basket 2 to Zone 2 of the Ninja Foodi 2-Basket Air Fryer.
8. Choose the "Air Fry" mode for Zone 1 at 350 degrees F and 9 minutes of cooking time.
9. Select the "MATCH COOK" option to copy the settings for Zone 2.
10. Initiate cooking by pressing the START/PAUSE BUTTON.
11. Flip the skewers once cooked halfway through.
12. Serve warm.

Nutrition Info:
- (Per serving) Calories 546 | Fat 33.1g |Sodium 1201mg | Carbs 30g | Fiber 2.4g | Sugar 9.7g | Protein 32g

Chicken Vegetable Skewers

Servings: 6
Cooking Time: 15 Minutes
Ingredients:
- 900g chicken breasts, cubed
- 1 bell pepper, chopped
- 51g Swerve
- 1 tsp ginger, grated
- 350g zucchini, chopped
- 8 mushrooms, sliced
- ½ medium onion, chopped
- 6 garlic cloves, crushed
- 120ml soy sauce

Directions:
1. Add chicken and the remaining ingredients to a zip-lock bag. Seal the bag and place it in the refrigerator overnight.
2. Thread the marinated chicken, zucchini, mushrooms, onion, and bell pepper onto the skewers.
3. Insert a crisper plate in the Ninja Foodi air fryer baskets.
4. Place skewers in both baskets.
5. Select zone 1 then select "air fry" mode and set the temperature to 380 degrees F for 15 minutes. Press "match" to match zone 2 settings to zone 1. Press "start/stop" to begin.

Nutrition Info:
- (Per serving) Calories 329 | Fat 11.5g |Sodium 1335mg | Carbs 8.6g | Fiber 1.4g | Sugar 2.9g | Protein 46.8g

Chicken And Broccoli

Servings: 4
Cooking Time: 15 Minutes
Ingredients:
- 1-pound boneless, skinless chicken breast or thighs, cut into 1-inch bite-sized pieces
- ¼ –½ pound broccoli, cut into florets (1–2 cups)
- ½ medium onion, cut into thick slices
- 3 tablespoons olive oil or grape seed oil
- ½ teaspoon garlic powder
- 1 tablespoon fresh minced ginger
- 1 tablespoon low-sodium soy sauce
- 1 tablespoon rice vinegar
- 1 teaspoon sesame oil
- 2 teaspoons hot sauce (optional)
- ½ teaspoon sea salt, or to taste
- Black pepper, to taste
- Lemon wedges, for serving (optional)

Directions:
1. Combine the oil, garlic powder, ginger, soy sauce, rice vinegar, sesame oil, optional spicy sauce, salt, and pepper in a large mixing bowl.
2. Put the chicken in a separate bowl.
3. In a separate bowl, combine the broccoli and onions.
4. Divide the marinade between the two bowls and toss to evenly coat each.
5. Install a crisper plate into both drawers. Place the broccoli in the zone 1 drawer, then insert the drawer into the unit. Place the chicken breasts in the zone 2 drawer, then insert the drawer into the unit.
6. Select zone 1, select AIR FRY, set temperature to 390 degrees F/ 200 degrees C, and set time to 10 minutes. Select zone 2, select AIR FRY, set temperature to 390 degrees F/ 200 degrees C, and set time to 20 minutes. Select SYNC. Press the START/STOP button to begin cooking.
7. When zone 2 time reaches 9 minutes, press START/STOP to pause the unit. Remove the drawer and toss the chicken. Re-insert the drawer into the unit and press START/STOP to resume cooking.
8. When cooking is complete, serve the chicken breasts and broccoli while still hot.
9. Add additional salt and pepper to taste. Squeeze optional fresh lemon juice on top and serve warm.

Nutrition Info:
- (Per serving) Calories 224 | Fat 15.8g | Sodium 203mg | Carbs 4g | Fiber 1g | Sugar 1g | Protein 25g

Chicken & Broccoli

Servings: 4
Cooking Time: 20 Minutes
Ingredients:
- 450g chicken breasts, boneless & cut into 1-inch pieces
- 1 tsp sesame oil
- 15ml soy sauce
- 1 tsp garlic powder
- 45ml olive oil
- 350g broccoli florets
- 2 tsp hot sauce
- 2 tsp rice vinegar
- Pepper
- Salt

Directions:
1. In a bowl, add chicken, broccoli florets, and remaining ingredients and mix well.

2. Insert a crisper plate in the Ninja Foodi air fryer baskets.
3. Add the chicken and broccoli mixture in both baskets.
4. Select zone 1, then select "air fry" mode and set the temperature to 380 degrees F for 20 minutes. Press "match" and press "start/stop" to begin.

Nutrition Info:
- (Per serving) Calories 337 | Fat 20.2g |Sodium 440mg | Carbs 3.9g | Fiber 1.3g | Sugar 1g | Protein 34.5g

Chicken And Potatoes

Servings: 2
Cooking Time: 10 Minutes
Ingredients:
- 2 potatoes, diced
- 2 chicken breasts, diced
- 4 cloves garlic crushed
- 2 teaspoons smoked paprika
- ½ teaspoon red chili flakes
- 1 teaspoon fresh thyme
- 1 teaspoon salt
- ¼ teaspoon black pepper
- 2 tablespoons olive oil

Directions:
1. Rub chicken with half of the salt, black pepper, oil, thyme, red chili flakes, paprika and garlic.
2. Mix potatoes with remaining spices, oil and garlic in a bowl.
3. Add chicken to one air fryer basket and potatoes the second basket.
4. Return the air fryer basket 1 to Zone 1, and basket 2 to Zone 2 of the Ninja Foodi 2-Basket Air Fryer.
5. Choose the "Air Fry" mode for Zone 1 at 375 degrees F and 10 minutes of cooking time.
6. Select the "MATCH COOK" option to copy the settings for Zone 2.
7. Initiate cooking by pressing the START/PAUSE BUTTON.
8. Flip the chicken and toss potatoes once cooked halfway through.
9. Garnish with chopped parsley.
10. Serve chicken with the potatoes.

Nutrition Info:
- (Per serving) Calories 374 | Fat 13g |Sodium 552mg | Carbs 25g | Fiber 1.2g | Sugar 1.2g | Protein 37.7g

Crispy Sesame Chicken

Servings: 2
Cooking Time: 10 Minutes
Ingredients:
- 680g boneless chicken thighs, diced
- 2 tablespoons rice vinegar
- 1 tablespoon soy sauce
- 2 teaspoons minced fresh ginger
- 1 garlic clove, minced
- ¾ teaspoon salt
- ½ teaspoon black pepper
- 2 large eggs, beaten
- 1 cup cornstarch
- Sauce
- 59ml soy sauce
- 2 tablespoons rice vinegar
- ⅓ cup brown sugar
- 59ml water
- 1 tablespoon cornstarch
- 2 teaspoons sesame oil
- 2 tablespoons vegetable oil
- 2 garlic cloves, minced
- 2 teaspoons chile paste
- Garnish
- 1 tablespoon toasted sesame seeds

Directions:
1. Blend all the sauce ingredients in a saucepan and cook until it thickens then allow it to cool.
2. Mix chicken with black pepper, salt, garlic, ginger, vinegar, and soy sauce in a bowl.
3. Cover and marinate the chicken for 20 minutes.
4. Divide the chicken in the air fryer baskets.
5. Return the air fryer basket 1 to Zone 1, and basket 2 to Zone 2 of the Ninja Foodi 2-Basket Air Fryer.
6. Choose the "Air Fry" mode for Zone 1 and set the temperature to 400 degrees F and 10 minutes of cooking time.
7. Select the "MATCH COOK" option to copy the settings for Zone 2.
8. Initiate cooking by pressing the START/PAUSE BUTTON.
9. Pour the prepared sauce over the air fried chicken and drizzle sesame seeds on top.
10. Serve warm.

Nutrition Info:
- (Per serving) Calories 351 | Fat 16g |Sodium 777mg | Carbs 26g | Fiber 4g | Sugar 5g | Protein 28g

Lemon Chicken Thighs

Servings: 4
Cooking Time: 25 Minutes
Ingredients:
- ¼ cup butter, softened
- 3 garlic cloves, minced
- 2 teaspoons minced fresh rosemary or ½ teaspoon crushed dried rosemary
- 1 teaspoon minced fresh thyme or ¼ teaspoon dried thyme
- 1 teaspoon grated lemon zest
- 1 tablespoon lemon juice
- 4 bone-in chicken thighs (about 1½ pounds)
- 1/8 teaspoon salt
- 1/8 teaspoon pepper

Directions:
1. Combine the butter, garlic, rosemary, thyme, lemon zest, and lemon juice in a small bowl.
2. Under the skin of each chicken thigh, spread 1 teaspoon of the butter mixture. Apply the remaining butter to each thigh's skin. Season to taste with salt and pepper.
3. Install a crisper plate in both drawers. Place half the chicken tenders in the zone 1 drawer and half in zone 2's, then insert the drawers into the unit.
4. Select zone 1, select AIR FRY, set temperature to 390 degrees F/ 200 degrees C, and set time to 22 minutes. Select MATCH to match zone 2 settings to zone 1. Press the START/STOP button to begin cooking.
5. When the time reaches 11 minutes, press START/STOP to pause the unit. Remove the drawers and flip the chicken. Re-insert the drawers into the unit and press START/STOP to resume cooking.
6. When cooking is complete, remove the chicken and serve.

Nutrition Info:
- (Per serving) Calories 329 | Fat 26g | Sodium 253mg | Carbs 1g | Fiber 0g | Sugar 0g | Protein 23g

Chicken Breast Strips

Servings:2
Cooking Time:22
Ingredients:
- 2 large organic egg
- 1-ounce buttermilk
- 1 cup of cornmeal
- ¼ cup all-purpose flour
- Salt and black pepper, to taste
- 1 pound of chicken breasts, cut into strips
- 2 tablespoons of oil bay seasoning
- oil spray, for greasing

Directions:
1. Take a medium bowl and whisk eggs with buttermilk.
2. In a separate large bowl mix flour, cornmeal, salt, black pepper, and oil bay seasoning.
3. First, dip the chicken breast strip in egg wash and then dredge into the flour mixture.
4. Coat the strip all over and layer on both the baskets that are already grease with oil spray.
5. Grease the chicken breast strips with oil spray as well.
6. Set the zone 1 basket to AIR FRY mode at 400 degrees F for 22 minutes.
7. Select the MATCH button for zone 2.
8. Hit the start button to let the cooking start.
9. Once the cooking cycle is done, serve.

Nutrition Info:
- (Per serving) Calories 788| Fat25g| Sodium835 mg | Carbs60g | Fiber 4.9g| Sugar1.5g | Protein79g

Desserts Recipes

Fried Dough With Roasted Strawberries

Servings: 4
Cooking Time: 20 Minutes
Ingredients:
- FOR THE FRIED DOUGH
- 6 ounces refrigerated pizza dough, at room temperature
- 2 tablespoons all-purpose flour, for dusting
- 4 tablespoons vegetable oil
- 2 tablespoons powdered sugar
- FOR THE ROASTED STRAWBERRIES
- 2 cups frozen whole strawberries
- 2 tablespoons granulated sugar

Directions:
1. To prep the fried dough: Divide the dough into four equal portions.
2. Dust a clean work surface with the flour. Place one dough portion on the surface and use a rolling pin to roll to a ⅛-inch thickness. Rub both sides of the dough with 1 tablespoon of oil. Repeat with remaining dough portions and oil.
3. To prep the strawberries: Place the strawberries in the Zone 2 basket. Sprinkle the granulated sugar on top.
4. To cook the fried dough and strawberries: Install a crisper plate in the Zone 1 basket. Place 2 dough portions in the basket and insert the basket in the unit. Insert the Zone 2 basket in the unit.
5. Select Zone 1, select AIR FRY, set the temperature to 400°F, and set the timer to 18 minutes.
6. Select Zone 2, select ROAST, set the temperature to 330°F, and set the timer to 20 minutes. Select SMART FINISH.
7. Press START/PAUSE to begin cooking.
8. When both timers read 8 minutes, press START/PAUSE. Remove the Zone 1 basket and transfer the fried dough to a cutting board. Place the 2 remaining dough portions in the basket, then reinsert the basket. Remove the Zone 2 basket and stir the strawberries. Reinsert the basket and press START/PAUSE to resume cooking.
9. When cooking is complete, the dough should be cooked through and the strawberries soft and jammy.
10. Sprinkle the fried dough with powdered sugar. Gently mash the strawberries with a fork. Spoon the strawberries onto each fried dough portion and serve.

Nutrition Info:
- (Per serving) Calories: 304; Total fat: 15g; Saturated fat: 2.5g; Carbohydrates: 38g; Fiber: 0.5g; Protein: 3g; Sodium: 421mg

Baked Apples

Servings: 4
Cooking Time: 15 Minutes
Ingredients:
- 4 apples
- 6 teaspoons raisins
- 2 teaspoons chopped walnuts
- 2 teaspoons honey
- ½ teaspoon cinnamon

Directions:
1. Chop off the head of the apples and scoop out the flesh from the center.
2. Stuff the apples with raisins, walnuts, honey and cinnamon.
3. Place these apples in the air fryer basket 1.
4. Return the air fryer basket 1 to Zone 1 of the Ninja Foodi 2-Basket Air Fryer.
5. Choose the "Air Fry" mode for Zone 1 and set the temperature to 350 degrees F and 15 minutes of cooking time.
6. Initiate cooking by pressing the START/PAUSE BUTTON.
7. Serve.

Nutrition Info:
- (Per serving) Calories 175 | Fat 13.1g | Sodium 154mg | Carbs 14g | Fiber 0.8g | Sugar 8.9g | Protein 0.7g

Banana Spring Rolls With Hot Fudge Dip

Servings: 4
Cooking Time: 10 Minutes
Ingredients:
- FOR THE BANANA SPRING ROLLS
- 1 large banana
- 4 egg roll wrappers
- 4 teaspoons light brown sugar
- Nonstick cooking spray
- FOR THE HOT FUDGE DIP
- ¼ cup sweetened condensed milk
- 2 tablespoons semisweet chocolate chips
- 1 tablespoon unsweetened cocoa powder
- 1 tablespoon unsalted butter
- ⅛ teaspoon kosher salt
- ⅛ teaspoon vanilla extract

Directions:
1. To prep the banana spring rolls: Peel the banana and halve it crosswise. Cut each piece in half lengthwise, for a total of 4 pieces.
2. Place one piece of banana diagonally across an egg roll wrapper. Sprinkle with 1 teaspoon of brown sugar. Fold the edges of the egg roll wrapper over the ends of

the banana, then roll to enclose the banana inside. Brush the edge of the wrapper with water and press to seal. Spritz with cooking spray. Repeat with the remaining bananas, egg roll wrappers, and brown sugar.
3. To prep the hot fudge dip: In an ovenproof ramekin or bowl, combine the condensed milk, chocolate chips, cocoa powder, butter, salt, and vanilla.
4. To cook the spring rolls and hot fudge dip: Install a crisper plate in each of the two baskets. Place the banana spring rolls seam-side down in the Zone 1 basket and insert the basket in the unit. Place the ramekin in the Zone 2 basket and insert the basket in the unit.
5. Select Zone 1, select AIR FRY, set the temperature to 390°F, and set the timer to 10 minutes.
6. Select Zone 2, select BAKE, set the temperature to 330°F, and set the timer to 8 minutes. Select SMART FINISH.
7. Press START/PAUSE to begin cooking.
8. When the Zone 2 timer reads 3 minutes, press START/PAUSE. Remove the basket and stir the hot fudge until smooth. Reinsert the basket and press START/PAUSE to resume cooking.
9. When cooking is complete, the spring rolls should be crisp.
10. Let the hot fudge cool for 2 to 3 minutes. Serve the banana spring rolls with hot fudge for dipping.
Nutrition Info:
- (Per serving) Calories: 268; Total fat: 10g; Saturated fat: 4g; Carbohydrates: 42g; Fiber: 2g; Protein: 5g; Sodium: 245mg

Monkey Bread

Servings: 12
Cooking Time: 10 Minutes
Ingredients:
- Bread
- 12 Rhodes white dinner rolls
- ½ cup brown sugar
- 1 teaspoon cinnamon
- 4 tablespoons butter melted
- Glaze
- ½ cup powdered sugar
- 1-2 tablespoons milk
- ½ teaspoon vanilla

Directions:
1. Mix brown sugar, cinnamon and butter in a bowl.
2. Cut the dinner rolls in half and dip them in the sugar mixture.
3. Place these buns in a greased baking pan and pour the remaining butter on top.
4. Place the buns in the air fryer baskets.
5. Return the air fryer basket 1 to Zone 1, and basket 2 to Zone 2 of the Ninja Foodi 2-Basket Air Fryer.
6. Choose the "Air Fry" mode for Zone 1 at 350 degrees F and 10 minutes of cooking time.
7. Initiate cooking by pressing the START/PAUSE BUTTON.
8. Flip the rolls once cooked halfway through.
9. Meanwhile, mix milk, vanilla and sugar in a bowl.
10. Pour the glaze over the air fried rolls.
11. Serve.

Nutrition Info:
- (Per serving) Calories 192 | Fat 9.3g | Sodium 133mg | Carbs 27.1g | Fiber 1.4g | Sugar 19g | Protein 3.2g

Fudge Brownies

Servings: 4
Cooking Time: 16
Ingredients:
- 1/2 cup all-purpose flour
- 1/4 cup unsweetened cocoa powder
- 3/4 teaspoon kosher salt
- 2 large eggs, whisked
- 1 tablespoon almond milk
- 1/2 cup brown sugar
- 1/2 cup packed white sugar
- 1/2 tablespoon vanilla extract
- 8 ounces of semisweet chocolate chips, melted
- 2/4 cup unsalted butter, melted

Directions:
1. Take a medium bowl, and use a hand beater to whisk together eggs, milk, both the sugars and vanilla.
2. In a separate microwave-safe bowl, mix melted butter and chocolate and microwave it for 30 seconds to melt the chocolate.
3. Add all the listed dry ingredients to the chocolate mixture.
4. Now incorporate the egg bowl ingredient into the batter.
5. Spray a reasonable size round baking pan that fits in baskets of air fryer.
6. Grease the pan with cooking spray.
7. Now pour the batter into the pan, put the crisper plate in baskets.
8. Add the pans and insert the basket into the unit.
9. Select the AIR FRY mode and adjust the setting the temperature to 300 degrees F, for 30 minutes.
10. Check it after 35 minutes and if not done, cook for 10 more minutes
11. Once it's done, take it out and let it get cool before serving.
12. Enjoy.

Nutrition Info:
- (Per serving) Calories 760| Fat43.3 g| Sodium644 mg | Carbs 93.2g | Fiber5.3 g | Sugar 70.2g | Protein 6.2g

Chocolate Chip Cake

Servings: 4
Cooking Time: 15
Ingredients:
- Salt, pinch
- 2 eggs, whisked
- ½ cup brown sugar
- ½ cup butter, melted
- 10 tablespoons of almond milk
- ¼ teaspoon of vanilla extract
- ½ teaspoon of baking powder
- 1 cup all-purpose flour
- 1 cup of chocolate chips
- ½ cup of cocoa powder

Directions:
1. Take 2 round baking pan that fits inside the baskets of the air fryer.
2. layer it with baking paper, cut it to the size of a baking pan.
3. In a bowl, whisk the egg, brown sugar, butter, almond milk, and vanilla extract.
4. Whisk it all very well with an electric hand beater.
5. In a second bowl, mix the flour, cocoa powder, baking powder, and salt.
6. Now, mix the dry ingredients slowly with the wet ingredients.
7. Now, at the end fold in the chocolate chips.
8. Incorporate all the ingredients well.
9. Divide this batter into the round baking pan.
10. Set the time for zone 1 to 16 minutes at 350 degrees F at AIR FRY mode.
11. Select the MATCH button for the zone 2 baskets.
12. Check if not done, and let it AIR FRY for one more minute.
13. Once it is done, serve.

Nutrition Info:
- (Per serving) Calories 736| Fat 45.5g| Sodium 356mg | Carbs 78.2g | Fiber 6.1g | Sugar 32.7g | Protein 11.5 g

Chocolate Cookies

Servings: 18
Cooking Time: 7 Minutes
Ingredients:
- 96g flour
- 57g butter, softened
- 15ml milk
- 7.5g cocoa powder
- 80g chocolate chips
- ½ tsp vanilla
- 35g sugar
- ¼ tsp baking soda
- Pinch of salt

Directions:
1. In a bowl, mix flour, cocoa powder, sugar, baking soda, vanilla, butter, milk, and salt until well combined.
2. Add chocolate chips and mix well.
3. Insert a crisper plate in Ninja Foodi air fryer baskets.
4. Make cookies from the mixture and place in both baskets.
5. Select zone 1 then select "air fry" mode and set the temperature to 360 degrees F for 7 minutes. Press "match" to match zone 2 settings to zone 1. Press "start/stop" to begin.

Nutrition Info:
- (Per serving) Calories 82 | Fat 4.1g |Sodium 47mg | Carbs 10.7g | Fiber 0.4g | Sugar 6.2g | Protein 1g

Mini Strawberry And Cream Pies

Servings: 2
Cooking Time: 10
Ingredients:
- 1 box Store-Bought Pie Dough, Trader Joe's
- 1 cup strawberries, cubed
- 3 tablespoons of cream, heavy
- 2 tablespoons of almonds
- 1 egg white, for brushing

Directions:
1. Take the store brought pie dough and flatten it on a surface.
2. Use a round cutter to cut it into 3-inch circles.
3. Brush the dough with egg white all around the parameters.
4. Now add almonds, strawberries, and cream in a very little amount in the center of the dough, and top it with another circular.
5. Press the edges with the fork to seal it.
6. Make a slit in the middle of the dough and divide it into the baskets.
7. Set zone 1 to AIR FRY mode 360 degrees for 10 minutes.
8. Select MATCH for zone 2 basket.
9. Once done, serve.

Nutrition Info:
- (Per serving) Calories 203| Fat 12.7g| Sodium 193mg | Carbs 20 g | Fiber 2.2g | Sugar 5.8g | Protein 3.7g

Bread Pudding

Servings: 4
Cooking Time: 15 Minutes
Ingredients:
- 2 cups bread cubes
- 1 egg
- ⅔ cup heavy cream
- ½ teaspoon vanilla extract
- ¼ cup sugar
- ¼ cup chocolate chips

Directions:

1. Grease two 4 inches baking dish with a cooking spray.
2. Divide the bread cubes in the baking dishes and sprinkle chocolate chips on top.
3. Beat egg with cream, sugar and vanilla in a bowl.
4. Divide this mixture in the baking dishes.
5. Place one pan in each air fryer basket.
6. Return the air fryer basket 1 to Zone 1, and basket 2 to Zone 2 of the Ninja Foodi 2-Basket Air Fryer.
7. Choose the "Air Fry" mode for Zone 1 at 350 degrees F and 15 minutes of cooking time.
8. Select the "MATCH COOK" option to copy the settings for Zone 2.
9. Initiate cooking by pressing the START/PAUSE BUTTON.
10. Allow the pudding to cool and serve.

Nutrition Info:
- (Per serving) Calories 149 | Fat 1.2g |Sodium 3mg | Carbs 37.6g | Fiber 5.8g | Sugar 29g | Protein 1.1g

Pumpkin Hand Pies Blueberry Hand Pies

Servings:4
Cooking Time: 15 Minutes
Ingredients:
- FOR THE PUMPKIN HAND PIES
- ½ cup pumpkin pie filling (from a 15-ounce can)
- ⅓ cup half-and-half
- 1 large egg
- ½ refrigerated pie crust (from a 14.1-ounce package)
- 1 large egg yolk
- 1 tablespoon whole milk
- FOR THE BLUEBERRY HAND PIES
- ¼ cup blueberries
- 2 tablespoons granulated sugar
- 1 tablespoon grated lemon zest (optional)
- ¼ teaspoon cornstarch
- 1 teaspoon fresh lemon juice
- ⅛ teaspoon kosher salt
- ½ refrigerated pie crust (from a 14.1-ounce package)
- 1 large egg yolk
- 1 tablespoon whole milk
- ½ teaspoon turbinado sugar

Directions:
1. To prep the pumpkin hand pies: In a small bowl, mix the pumpkin pie filling, half-and-half, and whole egg until well combined and smooth.
2. Cut the dough in half to form two wedges. Divide the pumpkin pie filling between the wedges. Fold the crust over to completely encase the filling. Using a fork, crimp the edges, forming a tight seal.
3. In a small bowl, whisk together the egg yolk and milk. Brush over the pastry. Carefully cut two small vents in the top of each pie.
4. To prep the blueberry hand pies: In a small bowl, combine the blueberries, granulated sugar, lemon zest (if using), cornstarch, lemon juice, and salt.
5. Cut the dough in half to form two wedges. Divide the blueberry filling between the wedges. Fold the crust over to completely encase the filling. Using a fork, crimp the edges, forming a tight seal.
6. In a small bowl, whisk together the egg yolk and milk. Brush over the pastry. Sprinkle with the turbinado sugar. Carefully cut two small vents in the top of each pie.
7. To cook the hand pies: Install a crisper plate in each of the two baskets. Place the pumpkin hand pies in the Zone 1 basket and insert the basket in the unit. Place the blueberry hand pies in the Zone 2 basket and insert the basket in the unit.
8. Select Zone 1, select AIR FRY, set the temperature to 350°F, and set the timer to 15 minutes. Select MATCH COOK to match Zone 2 settings to Zone 1.
9. Press START/PAUSE to begin cooking.
10. When cooking is complete, the pie crust should be crisp and golden brown and the filling bubbling.
11. Let the hand pies cool for at least 30 minutes before serving.

Nutrition Info:
- (Per serving) Calories: 588; Total fat: 33g; Saturated fat: 14g; Carbohydrates: 68g; Fiber: 0.5g; Protein: 10g; Sodium: 583mg

Zesty Cranberry Scones

Servings: 8
Cooking Time: 16 Minutes.
Ingredients:
- 4 cups of flour
- ½ cup brown sugar
- 2 tablespoons baking powder
- ½ teaspoon ground nutmeg
- ½ teaspoon salt
- ½ cup butter, chilled and diced
- 2 cups fresh cranberry
- ⅔ cup sugar
- 2 tablespoons orange zest
- 1 ¼ cups half and half cream
- 2 eggs

Directions:
1. Whisk flour with baking powder, salt, nutmeg, and both the sugars in a bowl.
2. Stir in egg and cream, mix well to form a smooth dough.
3. Fold in cranberries along with the orange zest.
4. Knead this dough well on a work surface.
5. Cut 3-inch circles out of the dough.
6. Divide the scones in the crisper plates and spray them with cooking oil.
7. Return the crisper plates to the Ninja Foodi Dual Zone Air Fryer.

8. Choose the Air Fry mode for Zone 1 and set the temperature to 375 degrees F and the time to 16 minutes.
9. Select the "MATCH" button to copy the settings for Zone 2.
10. Initiate cooking by pressing the START/STOP button.
11. Flip the scones once cooked halfway and resume cooking.
12. Enjoy!

Nutrition Info:
- (Per serving) Calories 204 | Fat 9g | Sodium 91mg | Carbs 27g | Fiber 2.4g | Sugar 15g | Protein 1.3g

Delicious Apple Fritters

Servings: 10
Cooking Time: 8 Minutes

Ingredients:
- 236g Bisquick
- 2 apples, peel & dice
- 158ml milk
- 30ml butter, melted
- 1 tsp cinnamon
- 24g sugar

Directions:
1. In a bowl, mix Bisquick, cinnamon, and sugar.
2. Add milk and mix until dough forms. Add apple and stir well.
3. Insert a crisper plate in Ninja Foodi air fryer baskets.
4. Make fritters from the mixture and place in both baskets. Brush fritters with melted butter.
5. Select zone 1 then select "air fry" mode and set the temperature to 360 degrees F for 10 minutes. Press "match" to match zone 2 settings to zone 1. Press "start/stop" to begin.

Nutrition Info:
- (Per serving) Calories 171 | Fat 6.7g | Sodium 352mg | Carbs 25.8g | Fiber 1.7g | Sugar 10.8g | Protein 2.7g

Air Fried Bananas

Servings: 4
Cooking Time: 13 Minutes.

Ingredients:
- 4 bananas, sliced
- 1 avocado oil cooking spray

Directions:
1. Spread the banana slices in the two crisper plates in a single layer.
2. Drizzle avocado oil over the banana slices.
3. Return the crisper plate to the Ninja Foodi Dual Zone Air Fryer.
4. Choose the Air Fry mode for Zone 1 and set the temperature to 350 degrees F and the time to 13 minutes.
5. Select the "MATCH" button to copy the settings for Zone 2.
6. Initiate cooking by pressing the START/STOP button.
7. Serve.

Nutrition Info:
- (Per serving) Calories 149 | Fat 1.2g | Sodium 3mg | Carbs 37.6g | Fiber 5.8g | Sugar 29g | Protein 1.1g

Strawberry Shortcake

Servings: 8
Cooking Time: 9 Minutes

Ingredients:
- Strawberry topping
- 1-pint strawberries sliced
- ½ cup confectioner's sugar substitute
- Shortcake
- 2 cups Carbquick baking biscuit mix
- ¼ cup butter cold, cubed
- ½ cup confectioner's sugar substitute
- Pinch salt
- ⅔ cup water
- Garnish: sugar free whipped cream

Directions:
1. Mix the shortcake ingredients in a bowl until smooth.
2. Divide the dough into 6 biscuits.
3. Place the biscuits in the air fryer basket 1.
4. Return the air fryer basket 1 to Zone 1 of the Ninja Foodi 2-Basket Air Fryer.
5. Choose the "Air Fry" mode for Zone 1 and set the temperature 400 degrees F and 9 minutes of cooking time.
6. Initiate cooking by pressing the START/PAUSE BUTTON.
7. Mix strawberries with sugar in a saucepan and cook until the mixture thickens.
8. Slice the biscuits in half and add strawberry sauce in between two halves of a biscuit.
9. Serve.

Nutrition Info:
- (Per serving) Calories 157 | Fat 1.3g | Sodium 27mg | Carbs 1.3g | Fiber 1g | Sugar 2.2g | Protein 8.2g

"air-fried" Oreos Apple Fries

Servings: 4
Cooking Time: 10 Minutes

Ingredients:
- FOR THE "FRIED" OREOS
- 1 teaspoon vegetable oil
- 1 cup all-purpose flour
- 1 tablespoon granulated sugar
- 1 tablespoon baking powder
- ½ teaspoon baking soda
- ¼ teaspoon kosher salt
- 1 large egg
- ¼ cup unsweetened almond milk

- ½ teaspoon vanilla extract
- 8 Oreo cookies
- Nonstick cooking spray
- 1 tablespoon powdered sugar (optional)
- FOR THE APPLE FRIES
- 1 teaspoon vegetable oil
- 1 cup all-purpose flour
- 1 tablespoon granulated sugar
- 1 tablespoon baking powder
- ½ teaspoon baking soda
- ¼ teaspoon kosher salt
- 1 large egg
- ¼ cup unsweetened almond milk
- ½ teaspoon vanilla extract
- 2 Granny Smith apples
- 2 tablespoons cornstarch
- ½ teaspoon apple pie spice
- Nonstick cooking spray
- 1 tablespoon powdered sugar (optional)

Directions:
1. To prep the "fried" Oreos: Brush a crisper plate with the oil and install it in the Zone 1 basket.
2. In a large bowl, combine the flour, granulated sugar, baking powder, baking soda, and salt. Mix in the egg, almond milk, and vanilla to form a thick batter.
3. Using a fork or slotted spoon, dip each cookie into the batter, coating it fully. Let the excess batter drip off, then place the cookies in the prepared basket in a single layer. Spritz each with cooking spray.
4. To prep the apple fries: Brush a crisper plate with the oil and install it in the Zone 2 basket.
5. In a large bowl, combine the flour, granulated sugar, baking powder, baking soda, and salt. Mix in the egg, almond milk, and vanilla to form a thick batter.
6. Core the apples and cut them into ½-inch-thick French fry shapes. Dust lightly with the cornstarch and apple pie spice.
7. Using a fork or slotted spoon, dip each apple into the batter, coating it fully. Let the excess batter drip off, then place the apples in the prepared basket in a single layer. Spritz with cooking spray.
8. To cook the "fried" Oreos and apple fries: Insert both baskets in the unit.
9. Select Zone 1, select AIR FRY, set the temperature to 400°F, and set the timer to 8 minutes.
10. Select Zone 2, select AIR FRY, set the temperature to 400°F, and set the timer to 10 minutes. Select SMART FINISH.
11. Press START/PAUSE to begin cooking.
12. When cooking is complete, the batter will be golden brown and crisp. If desired, dust the cookies and apples with the powdered sugar before serving.

Nutrition Info:
- (Per serving) Calories: 464; Total fat: 21g; Saturated fat: 3.5g; Carbohydrates: 66g; Fiber: 2.5g; Protein: 7g; Sodium: 293mg

Pumpkin Muffins

Servings:4
Cooking Time:20
Ingredients:
- 1 and ½ cups of all-purpose flour
- ½ teaspoon baking soda
- ½ teaspoon of baking powder
- 1 and 1/4 teaspoons cinnamon, groaned
- 1/4 teaspoon ground nutmeg, grated
- 2 large eggs
- Salt, pinch
- 3/4 cup granulated sugar
- 1/2 cup dark brown sugar
- 1 and 1/2 cups of pumpkin puree
- 1/4 cup coconut milk

Directions:
1. Take 4 ramekins that are the size of a cup and layer them with muffin papers.
2. Crack an egg in a bowl and add brown sugar, baking soda, baking powder, cinnamon, nutmeg, and sugar.
3. Whisk it all very well with an electric hand beater.
4. Now, in a second bowl, mix the flour, and salt.
5. Now, mix the dry ingredients slowly with the wet ingredients.
6. Now, at the end fold in the pumpkin puree and milk, mix it well
7. Divide this batter into 4 ramekins.
8. Now, divide ramekins between both zones.
9. Set the time for zone 1 to 18 minutes at 360 degrees Fat AIRFRY mode.
10. Select the MATCH button for the zone 2 basket.
11. Check if not done, and let it AIR FRY for one more minute.
12. Once it is done, serve.

Nutrition Info:
- (Per serving) Calories 291| Fat6.4 g| Sodium 241mg | Carbs 57.1g | Fiber 4.4g | Sugar42 g | Protein 5.9g

Mocha Pudding Cake Vanilla Pudding Cake

Servings:8
Cooking Time: 25 Minutes
Ingredients:
- FOR THE MOCHA PUDDING CAKE
- 1 cup all-purpose flour
- ⅔ cup granulated sugar
- 1 cup packed light brown sugar, divided
- 5 tablespoons unsweetened cocoa powder, divided
- 2 teaspoons baking powder
- ¼ teaspoon kosher salt
- ½ cup unsweetened almond milk
- 2 teaspoons vanilla extract
- 2 tablespoons vegetable oil

- 1 cup freshly brewed coffee
- FOR THE VANILLA PUDDING CAKE
- 1 cup all-purpose flour
- ⅔ cup granulated sugar, plus ½ cup
- 2 teaspoons baking powder
- ¼ teaspoon kosher salt
- ½ cup unsweetened almond milk
- 2½ teaspoons vanilla extract, divided
- 2 tablespoons vegetable oil
- ¾ cup hot water
- 2 teaspoons cornstarch

Directions:
1. To prep the mocha pudding cake: In a medium bowl, combine the flour, granulated sugar, ½ cup of brown sugar, 3 tablespoons of cocoa powder, the baking powder, and salt. Stir in the almond milk, vanilla, and oil to form a thick batter.
2. Spread the batter in the bottom of the Zone 1 basket. Sprinkle the remaining ½ cup brown sugar and 2 tablespoons of cocoa powder in an even layer over the batter. Gently pour the hot coffee over the batter (do not mix).
3. To prep the vanilla pudding cake: In a medium bowl, combine the flour, ⅔ cup of granulated sugar, the baking powder, and salt. Stir in the almond milk, 2 teaspoons of vanilla, and the oil to form a thick batter.
4. Spread the batter in the bottom of the Zone 2 basket.
5. In a small bowl, whisk together the hot water, cornstarch, and remaining ½ cup of sugar and ½ teaspoon of vanilla. Gently pour over the batter (do not mix).
6. To cook both pudding cakes: Insert both baskets in the unit.
7. Select Zone 1, select BAKE, set the temperature to 330°F, and set the timer to 25 minutes. Select MATCH COOK to match Zone 2 settings to Zone 1.
8. Press START/PAUSE to begin cooking.
9. When cooking is complete, the tops of the cakes should be dry and set.
10. Let the cakes rest for 10 minutes before serving. The pudding will thicken as it cools.

Nutrition Info:
- (Per serving) Calories: 531; Total fat: 8g; Saturated fat: 1g; Carbohydrates: 115g; Fiber: 3.5g; Protein: 5g; Sodium: 111mg

Healthy Semolina Pudding

Servings: 4
Cooking Time: 20 Minutes
Ingredients:
- 45g semolina
- 1 tsp vanilla
- 500ml milk
- 115g caster sugar

Directions:
1. Mix semolina and ½ cup milk in a bowl. Slowly add the remaining milk, sugar, and vanilla and mix well.
2. Pour the mixture into four greased ramekins.
3. Insert a crisper plate in the Ninja Foodi air fryer baskets.
4. Place ramekins in both baskets.
5. Select zone 1, then select "air fry" mode and set the temperature to 300 degrees F for 20 minutes. Press "match" to match zone 2 settings to zone 1. Press "start/stop" to begin.

Nutrition Info:
- (Per serving) Calories 209 | Fat 2.7g | Sodium 58mg | Carbs 41.5g | Fiber 0.6g | Sugar 30.6g | Protein 5.8g

Apple Crisp

Servings: 8
Cooking Time: 14 Minutes.
Ingredients:
- 3 cups apples, chopped
- 1 tablespoon pure maple syrup
- 2 teaspoons lemon juice
- 3 tablespoons all-purpose flour
- ⅓ cup quick oats
- ¼ cup brown sugar
- 2 tablespoons light butter, melted
- ½ teaspoon cinnamon

Directions:
1. Toss the chopped apples with 1 tablespoon of all-purpose flour, cinnamon, maple syrup, and lemon juice in a suitable bowl.
2. Divide the apples in the two air fryer baskets with their crisper plates.
3. Whisk oats, brown sugar, and remaining all-purpose flour in a small bowl.
4. Stir in melted butter, then divide this mixture over the apples.
5. Return the crisper plate to the Ninja Foodi Dual Zone Air Fryer.
6. Select the Bake mode for Zone 1 and set the temperature to 375 degrees F and the time to 14 minutes.
7. Select the "MATCH" button to copy the settings for Zone 2.
8. Initiate cooking by pressing the START/STOP button.
9. Enjoy fresh.

Nutrition Info:
- (Per serving) Calories 258 | Fat 12.4g | Sodium 79mg | Carbs 34.3g | Fiber 1g | Sugar 17g | Protein 3.2g

Dehydrated Peaches

Servings: 4
Cooking Time: 8 Hours
Ingredients:
- 300g canned peaches

Directions:
1. Insert a crisper plate in the Ninja Foodi air fryer baskets.
2. Place peaches in both baskets.
3. Select zone 1, then select "dehydrate" mode and set the temperature to 135 degrees F for 8 hours. Press "start/stop" to begin.

Nutrition Info:
- (Per serving) Calories 30 | Fat 0.2g |Sodium 0mg | Carbs 7g | Fiber 1.2g | Sugar 7g | Protein 0.7g

Pumpkin Muffins With Cinnamon

Servings: 4
Cooking Time: 20 Minutes
Ingredients:
- 1 and ½ cups all-purpose flour
- ½ teaspoon baking soda
- ½ teaspoon baking powder
- 1 and ¼ teaspoons cinnamon, groaned
- ¼ teaspoon ground nutmeg, grated
- 2 large eggs
- Salt, pinch
- ¾ cup granulated sugar
- ½ cup dark brown sugar
- 1 and ½ cups pumpkin puree
- ¼ cup coconut milk

Directions:
1. Take 4 ramekins and layer them with muffin paper.
2. In a bowl, add the eggs, brown sugar, baking soda, baking powder, cinnamon, nutmeg, and sugar and whisk well with an electric mixer.
3. In a second bowl, mix the flour, and salt.
4. Slowly add the dry ingredients to the wet ingredients.
5. Fold in the pumpkin puree and milk and mix it in well.
6. Divide this batter into 4 ramekins.
7. Place two ramekins in each air fryer basket.
8. Set the time for zone 1 to 18 minutes at 360 degrees F/ 180 degrees C on AIR FRY mode.
9. Select the MATCH button for the zone 2 basket.
10. Check after the time is up and if not done, and let it AIR FRY for one more minute.
11. Once it is done, serve.

Nutrition Info:
- (Per serving) Calories 291 | Fat 6.4g | Sodium 241mg | Carbs 57.1g | Fiber 4.4g | Sugar 42g | Protein 5.9g

Cinnamon Bread Twists

Servings: 4
Cooking Time: 15 Minutes
Ingredients:
- Bread Twists Dough
- 120g all-purpose flour
- 1 teaspoon baking powder
- ¼ teaspoon salt
- 150g fat free Greek yogurt
- Brushing
- 2 tablespoons light butter
- 2 tablespoons granulated sugar
- 1-2 teaspoons ground cinnamon, to taste

Directions:
1. Mix flour, salt and baking powder in a bowl.
2. Stir in yogurt and the rest of the dough ingredients in a bowl.
3. Mix well and make 8 inches long strips out of this dough.
4. Twist the strips and place them in the air fryer baskets.
5. Return the air fryer basket 1 to Zone 1, and basket 2 to Zone 2 of the Ninja Foodi 2-Basket Air Fryer.
6. Choose the "Air Fry" mode for Zone 1 at 375 degrees F and 15 minutes of cooking time.
7. Select the "MATCH COOK" option to copy the settings for Zone 2.
8. Initiate cooking by pressing the START/PAUSE BUTTON.
9. Flip the twists once cooked halfway through.
10. Mix butter with cinnamon and sugar in a bowl.
11. Brush this mixture over the twists.
12. Serve.

Nutrition Info:
- (Per serving) Calories 391 | Fat 24g |Sodium 142mg | Carbs 38.5g | Fiber 3.5g | Sugar 21g | Protein 6.6g

Chocó Lava Cake

Servings: 4
Cooking Time: 10 Minutes
Ingredients:
- 3 eggs
- 3 egg yolks
- 70g dark chocolate, chopped
- 168g cups powdered sugar
- 96g all-purpose flour
- 1 tsp vanilla
- 113g butter
- ½ tsp salt

Directions:
1. Add chocolate and butter to a bowl and microwave for 30 seconds. Remove from oven and stir until smooth.
2. Add eggs, egg yolks, sugar, flour, vanilla, and salt into the melted chocolate and stir until well combined.
3. Pour batter into the four greased ramekins.

4. Insert a crisper plate in Ninja Foodi air fryer baskets.
5. Place ramekins in both baskets.
6. Select zone 1 then select "air fry" mode and set the temperature to 390 degrees F for 10 minutes. Press "match" to match zone 2 settings to zone 1. Press "start/stop" to begin.

Nutrition Info:
- (Per serving) Calories 687 | Fat 37.3g |Sodium 527mg | Carbs 78.3g | Fiber 1.5g | Sugar 57.4g | Protein 10.7g

Moist Chocolate Espresso Muffins

Servings: 8
Cooking Time: 18 Minutes
Ingredients:
- 1 egg
- 177ml milk
- ½ tsp baking soda
- ½ tsp espresso powder
- ½ tsp baking powder
- 50g cocoa powder
- 78ml vegetable oil
- 1 tsp apple cider vinegar
- 1 tsp vanilla
- 150g brown sugar
- 150g all-purpose flour
- ½ tsp salt

Directions:
1. In a bowl, whisk egg, vinegar, oil, brown sugar, vanilla, and milk.
2. Add flour, cocoa powder, baking soda, baking powder, espresso powder, and salt and stir until well combined.
3. Pour batter into the silicone muffin moulds.
4. Insert a crisper plate in Ninja Foodi air fryer baskets.
5. Place muffin moulds in both baskets.
6. Select zone 1 then select "bake" mode and set the temperature to 320 degrees F for 18 minutes. Press match cook to match zone 2 settings to zone 1. Press "start/stop" to begin.

Nutrition Info:
- (Per serving) Calories 222 | Fat 11g |Sodium 251mg | Carbs 29.6g | Fiber 2g | Sugar 14.5g | Protein 4g

Walnut Baklava Bites Pistachio Baklava Bites

Servings:12
Cooking Time: 10 Minutes
Ingredients:
- FOR THE WALNUT BAKLAVA BITES
- ¼ cup finely chopped walnuts
- 2 teaspoons cold unsalted butter, grated
- 2 teaspoons granulated sugar
- ½ teaspoon ground cinnamon
- 6 frozen phyllo shells (from a 1.9-ounce package), thawed
- FOR THE PISTACHIO BAKLAVA BITES
- ¼ cup finely chopped pistachios
- 2 teaspoons very cold unsalted butter, grated
- 2 teaspoons granulated sugar
- ¼ teaspoon ground cardamom (optional)
- 6 frozen phyllo shells (from a 1.9-ounce package), thawed
- FOR THE HONEY SYRUP
- ¼ cup hot water
- ¼ cup honey
- 2 teaspoons fresh lemon juice

Directions:
1. To prep the walnut baklava bites: In a small bowl, combine the walnuts, butter, sugar, and cinnamon. Spoon the filling into the phyllo shells.
2. To prep the pistachio baklava bites: In a small bowl, combine the pistachios, butter, sugar, and cardamom (if using). Spoon the filling into the phyllo shells.
3. To cook the baklava bites: Install a crisper plate in each of the two baskets. Place the walnut baklava bites in the Zone 1 basket and insert the basket in the unit. Place the pistachio baklava bites in the Zone 2 basket and insert the basket in the unit.
4. Select Zone 1, select BAKE, set the temperature to 330°F, and set the timer to 10 minutes. Press MATCH COOK to match Zone 2 settings to Zone 1.
5. Press START/PAUSE to begin cooking.
6. When cooking is complete, the shells will be golden brown and crisp.
7. To make the honey syrup: In a small bowl, whisk together the hot water, honey, and lemon juice. Dividing evenly, pour the syrup over the baklava bites (you may hear a crackling sound).
8. Let cool completely before serving, about 1 hour.

Nutrition Info:
- (Per serving) Calories: 262; Total fat: 16g; Saturated fat: 3g; Carbohydrates: 29g; Fiber: 1g; Protein: 2g; Sodium: 39mg

Grilled Peaches

Servings: 2
Cooking Time: 5 Minutes
Ingredients:
- 2 yellow peaches, peeled and cut into wedges
- ¼ cup graham cracker crumbs
- ¼ cup brown sugar
- ¼ cup butter diced into tiny cubes
- Whipped cream or ice cream

Directions:
1. Toss peaches with crumbs, brown sugar, and butter in a bowl.
2. Spread the peaches in one air fryer basket.
3. Return the air fryer basket to the Ninja Foodi 2 Baskets Air Fryer.

4. Choose the "Air Fry" mode for Zone 1 and set the temperature to 350 degrees F and 5 minutes of cooking time.
5. Initiate cooking by pressing the START/PAUSE BUTTON.
6. Serve the peaches with a scoop of ice cream.

Nutrition Info:
- (Per serving) Calories 327 | Fat 14.2g |Sodium 672mg | Carbs 47.2g | Fiber 1.7g | Sugar 24.8g | Protein 4.4g

Apple Crumble Peach Crumble

Servings: 8
Cooking Time: 20 Minutes

Ingredients:
- FOR THE APPLE CRUMBLE
- ½ cup packed light brown sugar
- ¼ cup all-purpose flour
- ¼ cup rolled oats
- 2 tablespoons unsalted butter, at room temperature
- ½ teaspoon ground cinnamon
- ¼ teaspoon ground nutmeg
- ⅛ teaspoon kosher salt
- 4 medium Granny Smith apples, sliced
- FOR THE PEACH CRUMBLE
- ½ cup packed light brown sugar
- ¼ cup all-purpose flour
- ¼ cup rolled oats
- 2 tablespoons unsalted butter, at room temperature
- ½ teaspoon ground cinnamon
- ⅛ teaspoon kosher salt
- 4 peaches, peeled and sliced

Directions:
1. To prep the apple crumble: In a medium bowl, combine the brown sugar, flour, oats, butter, cinnamon, nutmeg, and salt and mix well. The mixture will be dry and crumbly.
2. To prep the peach crumble: In a medium bowl, combine the brown sugar, flour, oats, butter, cinnamon, and salt and mix well. The mixture will be dry and crumbly.
3. To cook both crumbles: Spread the apples in the Zone 1 basket in an even layer. Top evenly with the apple crumble topping and insert the basket in the unit. Spread the peaches in the Zone 2 basket in an even layer. Top with the peach crumble topping and insert the basket in the unit.
4. Select Zone 1, select BAKE, set the temperature to 350°F, and set the timer to 20 minutes. Select MATCH COOK to match Zone 2 settings to Zone 1.
5. Press START/PAUSE to begin cooking.
6. When cooking is complete, the fruit will be tender and the crumble topping crisp and golden brown. Serve warm or at room temperature.

Nutrition Info:
- (Per serving) Calories: 300; Total fat: 6.5g; Saturated fat: 3.5g; Carbohydrates: 59g; Fiber: 5.5g; Protein: 2g; Sodium: 45mg

Churros

Servings: 8
Cooking Time: 10 Minutes

Ingredients:
- 1 cup water
- ⅓ cup unsalted butter, cut into cubes
- 2 tablespoons granulated sugar
- ¼ teaspoon salt
- 1 cup all-purpose flour
- 2 large eggs
- 1 teaspoon vanilla extract
- Cooking oil spray
- For the cinnamon-sugar coating:
- ½ cup granulated sugar
- ¾ teaspoon ground cinnamon

Directions:
1. Add the water, butter, sugar, and salt to a medium pot. Bring to a boil over medium-high heat.
2. Reduce the heat to medium-low and stir in the flour. Cook, stirring constantly with a rubber spatula until the dough is smooth and comes together.
3. Remove the dough from the heat and place it in a mixing bowl. Allow 4 minutes for cooling.
4. In a mixing bowl, beat the eggs and vanilla extract with an electric hand mixer or stand mixer until the dough comes together. The finished product will resemble gluey mashed potatoes. Press the lumps together into a ball with your hands, then transfer to a large piping bag with a large star-shaped tip. Pipe out the churros.
5. Install a crisper plate in both drawers. Place half the churros in the zone 1 drawer and half in zone 2's, then insert the drawers into the unit.
6. Select zone 1, select AIR FRY, set temperature to 390 degrees F/ 200 degrees C, and set time to 12 minutes. Select MATCH to match zone 2 settings to zone 1. Press the START/STOP button to begin cooking.
7. In a shallow bowl, combine the granulated sugar and cinnamon.
8. Immediately transfer the baked churros to the bowl with the sugar mixture and toss to coat.

Nutrition Info:
- (Per serving) Calories 204 | Fat 9g | Sodium 91mg | Carbs 27g | Fiber 0.3g | Sugar 15g | Protein 3g

Apple Hand Pies

Servings: 8
Cooking Time: 21 Minutes.

Ingredients:
- 8 tablespoons butter, softened
- 12 tablespoons brown sugar
- 2 teaspoons cinnamon, ground

- 4 medium Granny Smith apples, diced
- 2 teaspoons cornstarch
- 4 teaspoons cold water
- 1 (14-oz) package pastry, 9-inch crust pie
- Cooking spray
- 1 tablespoon grapeseed oil
- ½ cup powdered sugar
- 2 teaspoons milk

Directions:
1. Toss apples with brown sugar, butter, and cinnamon in a suitable skillet.
2. Place the skillet over medium heat and stir cook for 5 minutes.
3. Mix cornstarch with cold water in a small bowl.
4. Add cornstarch mixture into the apple and cook for 1 minute until it thickens.
5. Remove this filling from the heat and allow it to cool.
6. Unroll the pie crust and spray on a floured surface.
7. Cut the dough into 16 equal rectangles.
8. Wet the edges of the 8 rectangles with water and divide the apple filling at the center of these rectangles.
9. Place the other 8 rectangles on top and crimp the edges with a fork, then make 2-3 slashes on top.
10. Place 4 small pics in each of the crisper plate.
11. Return the crisper plate to the Ninja Foodi Dual Zone Air Fryer.
12. Choose the Air Fry mode for Zone 1 and set the temperature to 390 degrees F and the time to 17 minutes.
13. Select the "MATCH" button to copy the settings for Zone 2.
14. Initiate cooking by pressing the START/STOP button.
15. Flip the pies once cooked halfway through, and resume cooking.
16. Meanwhile, mix sugar with milk.
17. Pour this mixture over the apple pies.
18. Serve fresh.

Nutrition Info:
- (Per serving) Calories 284 | Fat 16g |Sodium 252mg | Carbs 31.6g | Fiber 0.9g | Sugar 6.6g | Protein 3.7g

Air Fryer Sweet Twists

Servings: 2
Cooking Time: 9
Ingredients:
- 1 box store-bought puff pastry
- ½ teaspoon cinnamon
- ½ teaspoon sugar
- ½ teaspoon black sesame seeds
- Salt, pinch
- 2 tablespoons Parmesan cheese, freshly grated

Directions:
1. Place the dough on a work surface.
2. Take a small bowl and mix cheese, sugar, salt, sesame seeds, and cinnamon.
3. Press this mixture on both sides of the dough.
4. Now, cut the pastry into 1" x 3" strips.
5. Twist each of the strips 2 times and then lay it onto the flat.
6. Transfer to both the air fryer baskets.
7. Select zone 1 to air fry mode at 400 degrees F for 9-10 minutes.
8. Select the MATCH button for the zone 2 basket.
9. Once cooked, serve.

Nutrition Info:
- (Per serving) Calories 140| Fat 9.4g| Sodium 142mg | Carbs 12.3g | Fiber 0.8 g | Sugar 1.2g | Protein 2g

Dessert Empanadas

Servings: 12
Cooking Time: 10 Minutes
Ingredients:
- 12 empanada wrappers thawed
- 2 apples, chopped
- 2 tablespoons raw honey
- 1 teaspoon vanilla extract
- 1 teaspoon cinnamon
- ⅛ teaspoon nutmeg
- 2 teaspoons cornstarch
- 1 teaspoon water
- 1 egg beaten

Directions:
1. Mix apples with vanilla, honey, nutmeg, and cinnamon in a saucepan.
2. Cook for 3 minutes then mix cornstarch with water and pour into the pan.
3. Cook for 30 seconds.
4. Allow this filling to cool and keep it aside.
5. Spread the wrappers on the working surface.
6. Divide the apple filling on top of the wrappers.
7. Fold the wrappers in half and seal the edges by pressing them.
8. Brush the empanadas with the beaten egg and place them in the air fryer basket 1.
9. Return the air fryer basket 1 to Zone 1 of the Ninja Foodi 2-Basket Air Fryer.
10. Choose the "Air Fry" mode for Zone 1 at 400 degrees F and 10 minutes of cooking time.
11. Initiate cooking by pressing the START/PAUSE BUTTON.
12. Flip the empanadas once cooked halfway through.
13. Serve.

Nutrition Info:
- (Per serving) Calories 204 | Fat 9g |Sodium 91mg | Carbs 27g | Fiber 2.4g | Sugar 15g | Protein 1.3g

Lava Cake

Servings: 4
Cooking Time: 10 Minutes
Ingredients:
- 1 cup semi-sweet chocolate chips
- 8 tablespoons butter
- 4 eggs
- 2 teaspoons vanilla extract
- ½ teaspoon salt
- 6 tablespoons all-purpose flour
- 1 cup powdered sugar
- For the chocolate filling:
- 2 tablespoons Nutella
- 1 tablespoon butter, softened
- 1 tablespoon powdered sugar

Directions:
1. Heat the chocolate chips and butter in a medium-sized microwave-safe bowl in 30-second intervals until thoroughly melted and smooth, stirring after each interval.
2. Whisk together the eggs, vanilla, salt, flour, and powdered sugar in a mixing bowl.
3. Combine the Nutella, softened butter, and powdered sugar in a separate bowl.
4. Spray 4 ramekins with oil and fill them halfway with the chocolate chip mixture. Fill each ramekin halfway with Nutella, then top with the remaining chocolate chip mixture, making sure the Nutella is well covered.
5. Install a crisper plate in both drawers. Place 2 ramekins in each drawer and insert the drawers into the unit.
6. Select zone 1, select AIR FRY, set temperature to 390 degrees F/ 200 degrees C, and set time to 22 minutes. Select MATCH to match zone 2 settings to zone 1. Press the START/STOP button to begin cooking.
7. Serve hot.

Nutrition Info:
- (Per serving) Calories 338 | Fat 21.2g | Sodium 1503mg | Carbs 5.1g | Fiber 0.3g | Sugar 4.6g | Protein 29.3g

Apple Nutmeg Flautas

Servings: 8
Cooking Time: 8 Minutes.
Ingredients:
- ¼ cup light brown sugar
- ⅛ cup all-purpose flour
- ¼ teaspoon ground cinnamon
- Nutmeg, to taste
- 4 apples, peeled, cored & sliced
- ½ lemon, juice, and zest
- 6 (10-inch) flour tortillas
- Vegetable oil
- Caramel sauce
- Cinnamon sugar

Directions:
1. Mix brown sugar with cinnamon, nutmeg, and flour in a large bowl.
2. Toss in apples in lemon juice. Mix well.
3. Place a tortilla at a time on a flat surface and add ½ cup of the apple mixture to the tortilla.
4. Roll the tortilla into a burrito and seal it tightly and hold it in place with a toothpick.
5. Repeat the same steps with the remaining tortillas and apple mixture.
6. Place two apple burritos in each of the crisper plate and spray them with cooking oil.
7. Return the crisper plates to the Ninja Foodi Dual Zone Air Fryer.
8. Choose the Air Fry mode for Zone 1 and set the temperature to 400 degrees F and the time to 8 minutes.
9. Select the "MATCH" button to copy the settings for Zone 2.
10. Initiate cooking by pressing the START/STOP button.
11. Flip the burritos once cooked halfway through, then resume cooking.
12. Garnish with caramel sauce and cinnamon sugar.
13. Enjoy!

Nutrition Info:
- (Per serving) Calories 157 | Fat 1.3g | Sodium 27mg | Carbs 1.3g | Fiber 1g | Sugar 2.2g | Protein 8.2g

Jelly Donuts

Servings: 4
Cooking Time: 5 Minutes
Ingredients:
- 1 package Pillsbury Grands (Homestyle)
- ½ cup seedless raspberry jelly
- 1 tablespoon butter, melted
- ½ cup sugar

Directions:
1. Install a crisper plate in both drawers. Place half of the biscuits in the zone 1 drawer and half in zone 2's, then insert the drawers into the unit. You may need to cook in batches.
2. Select zone 1, select AIR FRY, set temperature to 390 degrees F/ 200 degrees C, and set time to 22 minutes. Select MATCH to match zone 2 settings to zone 1. Press the START/STOP button to begin cooking.
3. Place the sugar into a wide bowl with a flat bottom.
4. Baste all sides of the cooked biscuits with the melted butter and roll in the sugar to cover completely.
5. Using a long cake tip, pipe 1–2 tablespoons of raspberry jelly into each biscuit. You've now got raspberry-filled donuts!

Nutrition Info:
- (Per serving) Calories 252 | Fat 7g | Sodium 503mg | Carbs 45g | Fiber 0g | Sugar 23g | Protein 3g

Cinnamon Sugar Dessert Fries

Servings: 4
Cooking Time: 15 Minutes
Ingredients:
- 2 sweet potatoes
- 1 tablespoon butter, melted
- 1 teaspoon butter, melted
- 2 tablespoons sugar
- ½ teaspoon ground cinnamon

Directions:
1. Peel and cut the sweet potatoes into skinny fries.
2. Coat the fries with 1 tablespoon of butter.
3. Install a crisper plate into each drawer. Place half the sweet potatoes in the zone 1 drawer and half in zone 2's, then insert the drawers into the unit.
4. Select zone 1, select AIR FRY, set temperature to 390 degrees F/ 200 degrees C, and set time to 15 minutes. Select MATCH to match zone 2 settings to zone 1. Press the START/STOP button to begin cooking.
5. When the time reaches 11 minutes, press START/STOP to pause the unit. Remove the drawers and flip the fries. Re-insert the drawers into the unit and press START/STOP to resume cooking.
6. Meanwhile, mix the 1 teaspoon of butter, the sugar, and the cinnamon in a large bowl.
7. When the fries are done, add them to the bowl, and toss them to coat.
8. Serve and enjoy!

Nutrition Info:
- (Per serving) Calories 110 | Fat 4g | Sodium 51mg | Carbs 18g | Fiber 2g | Sugar 10g | Protein 1g

S'mores Dip With Cinnamon-sugar Tortillas

Servings: 4
Cooking Time: 5 Minutes
Ingredients:
- FOR THE S'MORES DIP
- ½ cup chocolate-hazelnut spread
- ¼ cup milk chocolate or white chocolate chips
- ¼ cup graham cracker crumbs
- ½ cup mini marshmallows
- FOR THE CINNAMON-SUGAR TORTILLAS
- 4 (6-inch) flour tortillas
- Butter-flavored cooking spray
- 1 teaspoon granulated sugar
- ½ teaspoon ground cinnamon
- ¼ teaspoon ground cardamom (optional)

Directions:
1. To prep the s'mores dip: Spread the chocolate-hazelnut spread in the bottom of a shallow ovenproof ramekin or dish.
2. Scatter the chocolate chips and graham cracker crumbs over the top. Arrange the marshmallows in a single layer on top of the crumbs.
3. To prep the tortillas: Spray both sides of each tortilla with cooking spray. Cut each tortilla into 8 wedges and sprinkle both sides evenly with sugar, cinnamon, and cardamom (if using).
4. To cook the dip and tortillas: Install a crisper plate in each of the two baskets. Place the ramekin in the Zone 1 basket and insert the basket in the unit. Place the tortillas in the Zone 2 basket and insert the basket in the unit.
5. Select Zone 1, select BAKE, set the temperature to 330°F, and set the timer to 5 minutes.
6. Select Zone 2, select AIR FRY, set the temperature to 375°F, and set the timer to 5 minutes. Select SMART FINISH.
7. Press START/PAUSE to begin cooking.
8. When the Zone 2 timer reads 3 minutes, press START/PAUSE. Remove the basket and shake it to redistribute the chips. Reinsert the basket and press START/PAUSE to resume cooking.
9. When cooking is complete, the dip will be bubbling and golden brown and the chips crispy.
10. If desired, toast the marshmallows more: Select Zone 1, select AIR BROIL, set the temperature to 450°F, and set the timer to 1 minute. Cook until the marshmallows are deep golden brown.
11. Let the dip cool for 2 to 3 minutes. Serve with the cinnamon-sugar tortilla chips.

Nutrition Info:
- (Per serving) Calories: 404; Total fat: 18g; Saturated fat: 7g; Carbohydrates: 54g; Fiber: 2.5g; Protein: 6g; Sodium: 346mg

APPENDIX A: Measurement

BASIC KITCHEN CONVERSIONS & EQUIVALENTS DRY MEASUREMENTS CONVERSION CHART

3 TEASPOONS = 1 TABLESPOON = 1/16 CUP

6 TEASPOONS = 2 TABLESPOONS = 1/8 CUP

12 TEASPOONS = 4 TABLESPOONS = 1/4 CUP

24 TEASPOONS = 8 TABLESPOONS = 1/2 CUP

36 TEASPOONS = 12 TABLESPOONS = 3/4 CUP

48 TEASPOONS = 16 TABLESPOONS = 1 CUP

METRIC TO US COOKING CONVERSIONS OVEN TEMPERATURES

120 ° C = 250 ° F 160 ° C = 320 ° F 180° C = 350 ° F 205 ° C = 400 ° F 220 ° C = 425 ° F

LIQUID MEASUREMENTS CONVERSION CHART

8 FLUID OUNCES = 1 CUP = 1/2 PINT = 1/4 QUART

16 FLUID OUNCES = 2 CUPS = 1 PINT = 1/2 QUART

32 FLUID OUNCES = 4 CUPS = 2 PINTS = 1 QUART = 1/4 GALLON

128 FLUID OUNCES = 16 CUPS = 8 PINTS = 4 QUARTS = 1 GALLON

BAKING IN GRAMS

1 CUP FLOUR = 140 GRAMS

1 CUP SUGAR = 150 GRAMS

1 CUP POWDERED SUGAR = 160 GRAMS

1 CUP HEAVY CREAM = 235 GRAMS

VOLUME

1 MILLILITER = 1/5 TEASPOON

5 ML = 1 TEASPOON

15 ML = 1 TABLESPOON

240 ML = 1 CUP OR 8 FLUID OUNCES

1 LITER = 34 FL. OUNCES

WEIGHT

1 GRAM = .035 OUNCES

100 GRAMS = 3.5 OUNCES

500 GRAMS = 1.1 POUNDS

1 KILOGRAM = 35 OUNCES

US TO METRIC COOKING CONVERSIONS

1/5 TSP = 1 ML

1 TSP = 5 ML

1 TBSP = 15 ML

1 FL OUNCE = 30 ML

1 CUP = 237 ML

1 PINT (2 CUPS) = 473 ML

1 QUART (4 CUPS) = .95 LITER

1 GALLON (16 CUPS) = 3.8 LITERS

1 OZ = 28 GRAMS

1 POUND = 454 GRAMS

BUTTER

1 CUP BUTTER = 2 STICKS = 8 OUNCES = 230 GRAMS = 8 TABLESPOONS

WHAT DOES 1 CUP EQUAL

1 CUP = 8 FLUID OUNCES

1 CUP = 16 TABLESPOONS

1 CUP = 48 TEASPOONS

1 CUP = 1/2 PINT

1 CUP = 1/4 QUART

1 CUP = 1/16 GALLON

1 CUP = 240 ML

BAKING PAN CONVERSIONS

1 CUP ALL-PURPOSE FLOUR = 4.5 OZ

1 CUP ROLLED OATS = 3 OZ 1 LARGE EGG = 1.7 OZ

1 CUP BUTTER = 8 OZ 1 CUP MILK = 8 OZ

1 CUP HEAVY CREAM = 8.4 OZ

1 CUP GRANULATED SUGAR = 7.1 OZ

1 CUP PACKED BROWN SUGAR = 7.75 OZ

1 CUP VEGETABLE OIL = 7.7 OZ

1 CUP UNSIFTED POWDERED SUGAR = 4.4 OZ

BAKING PAN CONVERSIONS

9-INCH ROUND CAKE PAN = 12 CUPS

10-INCH TUBE PAN = 16 CUPS

11-INCH BUNDT PAN = 12 CUPS

9-INCH SPRINGFORM PAN = 10 CUPS

9 X 5 INCH LOAF PAN = 8 CUPS

9-INCH SQUARE PAN = 8 CUPS

APPENDIX B: Recipes Index

A

"air-fried" Oreos Apple Fries 89
"fried" Chicken With Warm Baked Potato Salad 80
"fried" Ravioli With Zesty Marinara 30
Acorn Squash Slices 51
Air Fried Bananas 89
Air Fried Okra 48
Air Fried Sausage 15
Air Fryer Meatloaves 61
Air Fryer Sweet Twists 95
Air-fried Radishes 53
Air-fried Tofu Cutlets With Cacio E Pepe Brussels Sprouts 46
Air-fried Turkey Breast With Roasted Green Bean Casserole 77
Almond Chicken 76
Apple Crisp 91
Apple Crumble Peach Crumble 94
Apple Hand Pies 94
Apple Nutmeg Flautas 96
Asian Chicken 75

B

Bacon Potato Patties 53
Bacon Wrapped Corn Cob 51
Bacon Wrapped Pork Tenderloin 63
Bacon Wrapped Tater Tots 23
Bacon-wrapped Shrimp 38
Bagels 19
Baked Apples 85
Balsamic Duck Breast 73
Balsamic Steak Tips With Roasted Asparagus And Mushroom Medley 63
Banana And Raisins Muffins 19
Banana Muffins 13
Banana Spring Rolls With Hot Fudge Dip 85
Bang Bang Shrimp 41
Bang Bang Shrimp With Roasted Bok Choy 35
Bang-bang Chicken 76
Bbq Corn 57
Beef And Bean Taquitos With Mexican Rice 59
Beef Cheeseburgers 64
Beef Jerky Pineapple Jerky 25
Beef Ribs I 68
Beer Battered Fish Fillet 44
Bell Peppers With Sausages 62
Blueberries Muffins 27
Blueberry Coffee Cake And Maple Sausage Patties 14
Bread Pudding 87
Breaded Pork Chops 69
Breaded Scallops 34
Breakfast Bacon 22
Breakfast Frittata 15
Breakfast Sausage Omelet 20
Breakfast Stuffed Peppers 14
Broccoli, Squash, & Pepper 46
Brussels Sprouts Potato Hash 21
Buffalo Seitan With Crispy Zucchini Noodles 54
Buttered Mahi-mahi 37
Buttermilk Biscuits With Roasted Stone Fruit Compote 16
Buttermilk Fried Chicken 71

C

Cajun Chicken With Vegetables 80
Cajun Scallops 38
Cauliflower Gnocchi 23
Cheddar Quiche 24
Cheddar-stuffed Chicken 76
Cheesy Baked Eggs 18
Chicken & Broccoli 82
Chicken And Broccoli 82
Chicken And Potatoes 83
Chicken Breast Strips 84
Chicken Crescent Wraps 24
Chicken Drumettes 78
Chicken Kebabs 81
Chicken Parmesan With Roasted Lemon-parmesan Broccoli 72
Chicken Ranch Wraps 78
Chicken Vegetable Skewers 82
Chili Lime Tilapia 45
Chili-lime Crispy Chickpeas Pizza-seasoned Crispy Chickpeas 31
Chinese Bbq Pork 66
Chipotle Beef 70
Chocó Lava Cake 92
Chocolate Chip Cake 87
Chocolate Cookies 87
Churros 94
Cinnamon Apple French Toast 22
Cinnamon Bread Twists 92
Cinnamon Sugar Chickpeas 32
Cinnamon Sugar Dessert Fries 97
Cinnamon-apple Pork Chops 65
Coconut Chicken Tenders With Broiled Utica Greens 79
Codfish With Herb Vinaigrette 35
Cornbread 11
Cornish Hen With Asparagus 81
Crab Cakes 25
Crab Rangoon Dip With Crispy Wonton Strips 32
Crispy Catfish 35
Crispy Hash Browns 20
Crispy Plantain Chips 29
Crispy Sesame Chicken 83
Crusted Cod 44

Crusted Shrimp 37
Curly Fries 53

D

Dehydrated Peaches 92
Delicious Apple Fritters 89
Delicious Potatoes & Carrots 55
Dessert Empanadas 95
Dried Apple Chips Dried Banana Chips 33

E

Easy Breaded Pork Chops 60
Easy Chicken Thighs 78
Egg And Avocado In The Ninja Foodi 19
Egg White Muffins 16
Egg With Baby Spinach 17

F

Fish And Chips 38
Fish Tacos 45
Flavorful Salmon With Green Beans 40
Foil Packet Salmon 37
Fried Artichoke Hearts 52
Fried Asparagus 56
Fried Avocado Tacos 55
Fried Cheese 30
Fried Dough With Roasted Strawberries 85
Fried Halloumi Cheese 23
Fried Olives 57
Fried Patty Pan Squash 55
Fried Pickles 24
Fried Ravioli 28
Fried Tilapia 36
Frozen Breaded Fish Fillet 42
Fudge Brownies 86
Furikake Salmon 45

G

Garlic Butter Salmon 42
Garlic Butter Steaks 60
Garlic Potato Wedges In Air Fryer 56
Garlic-herb Fried Squash 56
Garlic-rosemary Brussels Sprouts 54
Garlic-rosemary Pork Loin With Scalloped Potatoes And Cauliflower 66
Glazed Apple Fritters Glazed Peach Fritters 21
Glazed Steak Recipe 68
Glazed Thighs With French Fries 74
Goat Cheese–stuffed Chicken Breast With Broiled Zucchini And Cherry Tomatoes 77
Gochujang Brisket 59
Greek Chicken Meatballs 79
Green Beans With Baked Potatoes 47

Green Tomato Stacks 52
Grilled Peaches 93

H

Hash Browns 18
Hasselback Potatoes 54
Healthy Air Fried Veggies 48
Healthy Oatmeal Muffins 11
Healthy Semolina Pudding 91
Healthy Spinach Balls 26
Herb Lemon Mussels 43
Herb Tuna Patties 41
Honey Banana Oatmeal 11
Honey Teriyaki Tilapia 41

I

Italian-style Meatballs With Garlicky Roasted Broccoli 63

J

Jelly Donuts 96
Jerk Tofu With Roasted Cabbage 46
Juicy Pork Chops 65

K

Kale And Spinach Chips 57
Kale Potato Nuggets 32
Korean Bbq Beef 67

L

Lamb Chops With Dijon Garlic 59
Lamb Shank With Mushroom Sauce 65
Lava Cake 96
Lemon Chicken Thighs 83
Lemon Pepper Fish Fillets 37
Lemon Pepper Salmon With Asparagus 40
Lemon-cream Cheese Danishes Cherry Danishes 12
Lime Glazed Tofu 49

M

Mac And Cheese Balls 29
Marinated Chicken Legs 75
Meatballs 62
Meatloaf 61
Mini Strawberry And Cream Pies 87
Miso-glazed Shishito Peppers Charred Lemon Shishito Peppers 27
Mixed Air Fry Veggies 51
Mocha Pudding Cake Vanilla Pudding Cake 90
Moist Chocolate Espresso Muffins 93
Monkey Bread 86

Morning Egg Rolls 17
Mozzarella Balls 31
Mushroom Roll-ups 57
Mustard Rubbed Lamb Chops 58

O
Onion Rings 26

P
Paprika Pork Chops 68
Parmesan Crush Chicken 33
Parmesan French Fries 26
Pepper Egg Cups 15
Peppered Asparagus 23
Perfect Cinnamon Toast 15
Pork Chops And Potatoes 68
Pork Chops With Apples 66
Pork Chops With Brussels Sprouts 64
Pork With Green Beans And Potatoes 62
Potato Chips 30
Potatoes & Beans 58
Pumpkin Hand Pies Blueberry Hand Pies 88
Pumpkin Muffins 90
Pumpkin Muffins With Cinnamon 92

Q
Quiche Breakfast Peppers 12
Quinoa Patties 49

R
Ranch Turkey Tenders With Roasted Vegetable Salad 71
Roast Beef 69
Roasted Garlic Chicken Pizza With Cauliflower "wings" 80
Roasted Tomato Bruschetta With Toasty Garlic Bread 33
Rosemary Asparagus & Potatoes 47

S
S'mores Dip With Cinnamon-sugar Tortillas 97
Salmon Nuggets 39
Salmon Patties 36
Salmon With Coconut 42
Sausage & Butternut Squash 18
Sausage Breakfast Casserole 20
Sausage Hash And Baked Eggs 13
Sausage Meatballs 69
Scallops With Greens 40
Seafood Shrimp Omelet 34
Shrimp Po'boys With Sweet Potato Fries 43
Shrimp With Lemon And Pepper 40
Smoked Salmon 43
Spanakopita Rolls With Mediterranean Vegetable Salad 48
Spice-rubbed Chicken Pieces 74
Spicy Chicken Sandwiches With "fried" Pickles 72
Spicy Chicken Tenders 24
Spicy Chicken Wings 73
Spicy Salmon Fillets 36
Steak Bites With Cowboy Butter 70
Steak In Air Fry 60
Strawberries And Walnuts Muffins 25
Strawberry Shortcake 89
Stuffed Bell Peppers 28
Stuffed Mushrooms With Crab 42
Stuffed Sweet Potatoes 47
Sweet And Spicy Carrots With Chicken Thighs 75
Sweet Bites 27
Sweet Potato Hash 13
Sweet Potato Sausage Hash 17
Sweet Potatoes & Brussels Sprouts 51
Sweet Potatoes Hash 14
Sweet-and-sour Chicken With Pineapple Cauliflower Rice 74

T
Tasty Pork Skewers 67
Tasty Sweet Potato Wedges 31
Tater Tots 29
Tender Pork Chops 64
Thai Curry Chicken Kabobs 76
Tilapia With Mojo And Crispy Plantains 39
Tofu Veggie Meatballs 28
Turkey And Beef Meatballs 61
Turkey Ham Muffins 20

V
Vanilla Strawberry Doughnuts 22
Veggie Burgers With "fried" Onion Rings 50

W
Walnut Baklava Bites Pistachio Baklava Bites 93
Wings With Corn On The Cob 73

Y
Yellow Potatoes With Eggs 11

Z
Zesty Cranberry Scones 88
Zucchini Cakes 52
Zucchini Chips 28

Printed in Great Britain
by Amazon

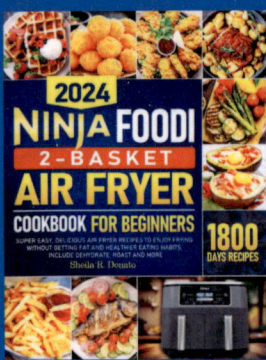

Ninja Foodi PossibleCooker Cookbook for Beginners 2024
1900 Days of Easy & Yummy Ninja Foodi PossibleCooker PRO Recipes to Enjoy Healthier Family Meals for Anyone |Including Slow Cook, Sear and More

2024 Ninja Foodi 2-Basket Air Fryer Cookbook: the secret to delicious, non-fattening food with 1,800 days of low-fat, crunchy air fryer dishes and more, so you can enjoy deep-frying and control your weight with ease!
 Harness the magic of the Ninja Foodi 2-Basket Air Fryer and shine!
 Explore the benefits of the air fryer diet
The Ninja Foodi 2-Basket Air Fryer not only gives you the freedom to achieve healthy fried meals at home, but also the versatility to cook, bake, dehydrate, Roast, and more, this recipe book for beginners is the perfect guide to adopt low-carb, low-oil cooking with ease!
 Dual-zone cooking for more efficiency
Ninja Foodi 2-Basket Air Fryer has two cooking baskets, you can choose to cook two different dishes at the same time according to your needs, which is more efficient and saves you more than half of your busy time in the kitchen
1800 easy dishes bursting with deliciousness
Superbly themed creative dishes for you to make again and again! There's never a shortage of culinary inspiration. Whether you're craving an appetizer, a main course, a side dish or a dessert, there are recipes for every occasion and taste. Every bite is a reward for your health and taste buds!

Enjoy every bite, and embark on a journey of simplified cooking with the Ninja Foodi 2-Basket Air Fryer Cook Book!

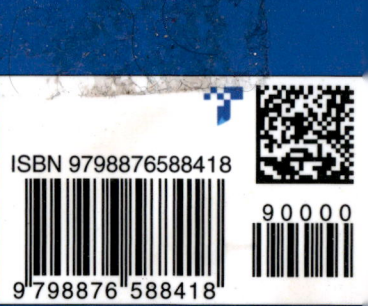